The Better Bladder Book

WENDY COHAN, a registered nurse for sixteen years, is an experienced health educator who counsels patients with celiac disease, non-celiac gluten intolerance, and bladder-related health conditions. Through sharing her personal story of recovery she promotes wider acceptance and knowledge of the link between gluten intolerance, urologic symptoms, and chronic pelvic pain. Wendy maintains the informational websites www.WellBladder .com and www.glutenfreechoice.com and consults privately with clients needing help transitioning to a gluten-free diet or those sorting through their treatment options for interstitial cystitis and overactive bladder.

Ms. Cohan also speaks publicly on gluten-related health issues, and, as a health writer, is a frequent contributor to www .celiac.com and other websites. Her first book, *Gluten-Free PORTLAND—A Resource Guide*, a comprehensive beginner's guide to the gluten-free diet, is available locally in the Northwest and through her website, www.glutenfreechoice.com.

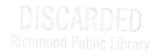

Ordering

Trade bookstores in the U.S. and Canada please contact:

Publishers Group West
1700 Fourth Street, Berkeley CA 94710
Phone: (800) 788-3123   Fax: (800) 351-5073

Hunter House books are available at bulk discounts for textbook course
adoptions; to qualifying community, health-care, and government organizations;
and for special promotions and fund-raising. For details please contact:

Special Sales Department
Hunter House Inc., PO Box 2914, Alameda CA 94501-0914
Phone: (510) 865-5282   Fax: (510) 865-4295
E-mail: ordering@hunterhouse.com

Individuals can order our books from most bookstores,
by calling **(800) 266-5592**, or from our website at
www.hunterhouse.com

The
Better
Bladder
Book

**A HOLISTIC
APPROACH
TO HEALING
INTERSTITIAL
CYSTITIS &
CHRONIC
PELVIC PAIN**

Wendy Cohan, RN

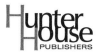

Hunter
House
PUBLISHERS

Hunter House Inc., Publishers
PO Box 2914
Alameda CA 94501-0914

Library of Congress Cataloging-in-Publication Data
Cohan, Wendy
The better bladder book : a holistic approach to healing interstitial cystitis and chronic pelvic pain / Wendy Cohan.
p.   cm.
Includes bibliographical references and index.
ISBN 978-0-89793-555-5
1. Interstitial cystitis—Popular works.   2. Interstitial cystitis—Alternative treatment—Popular works.   3. Bladder—Diseases—Diet therapy—Popular works.—I. Title.
RC921.C9C64 2010
616.6'2—dc22   2010006800

Project Credits

Cover Design: Stefanie Gold and Jinni Fonatana	Managing Editor: Alexandra Mummery
Book Production: John McKercher	Editorial Intern: Kelsey Comes
Illustrator: Leslie Anderson	Acquisitions Intern: Elizabeth Kracht
Developmental Editor: Jude Berman	Senior Marketing Associate: Reina Santana
Line and Copy Editor: Kelley Blewster	Publicity Coordinator: Sean Harvey
Proofreader: John David Marion	Rights Coordinator: Candace Groskreutz
Indexer: Candace Hyatt	Order Fulfillment: Washul Lakdhon
Computer Support: Peter Eichelberger	Administrator: Theresa Nelson
Customer Service Manager: Christina Sverdrup	
Publisher: Kiran S. Rana	

Printed and bound by Sheridan Books, Ann Arbor, Michigan
Manufactured in the United States of America

9 8 7 6 5 4 3 2   First Edition   11 12 13 14 15

Contents

**Part III: Further Along the Road to Recovery:
Suggestions for Those Who Are Still Struggling**

Foreword

by Dr. John Toth

Frustration is perhaps the most frequent complaint voiced by individuals who suffer from chronic pelvic pain. Frustration, not pain. Perhaps this is because many pelvic pain sufferers find it difficult to talk openly about their problem; they have suffered for so long, they fear their pain will never go away, and some of them feel that no one else could possibly understand what they are going through.

The Better Bladder Book is written from the perspective of a former IC patient who has devoted countless hours and extensive research to finding the answers sought by every pelvic pain sufferer. Through sheer determination, she has beaten the odds against recovery, and now she shares her healing journey with those who continue to suffer from interstitial cystitis and chronic pelvic pain.

This book is an invaluable resource for people dealing with this very private, very complex, and very common concern. Wendy Cohan, RN, has done a superb job bringing to light the many and varied factors comprising pelvic pain syndrome. More importantly, she has broken with the rather dated, traditional medical viewpoint that the cause of pelvic pain is often unknown, that it is an isolated entity, and that infection plays no part.

Furthermore, she sheds light on the growing body of evidence that indicates that interstitial cystitis is a systemic disease. Like the eye, the bladder can be utilized as a window through which to view a more comprehensive systemic process. Just as the eye is the body's window through which we can view early signs of systemic vascular disease, the bladder can often be the body's indicator of generalized inflammation and autoimmunity, sometimes making itself known through the occurrence of occult, or hidden, urinary tract infection.

The Better Bladder Book is a very readable text that broadens the readers' knowledge about a multifaceted disease complex while offering a wealth of natural solutions in a field overrun with drugs and invasive procedures.

— John Toth, DO
Associate of the late Paul Fugazzotto, PhD
Cystitis Research Center and Advanced Integrative Medicine
Concord, CA
http://drjohntoth.com

Foreword

by Dr. Lisa Shaver

Since you have found this book by Wendy Cohan, RN, chances are you will soon find relief among her many well-researched suggestions — relief from pelvic pain, as well as from the bladder symptoms that interrupt your daily activities and negatively affect your relationships, your ability to work, recreate, and enjoy life. More than a list of research-based tips, Wendy has created a guide that each person can apply *today* to start feeling better.

As a naturopathic physician and acupuncturist, I commend the gift Ms. Cohan has given those who are suffering from chronic pelvic pain. She has made a strong case for the urgent need to look at the body as a whole interconnected system that is inflamed and crying for help, versus focusing exclusively on the bladder tissue. Viewing the body holistically and finding the individual root cause of discomfort for each person, and effectively addressing that cause, is the path to health for each of us.

As a faculty instructor in histology (the study of organ tissues), I teach my medical students to look at the form and function of tissues of the bladder and urethra, with the ever-present philosophy that the *whole* body and the lifestyle choices we make affect each specific tissue of every organ. To look at the body systemically is essential to finding relief for any chronic condition, and Wendy has achieved this in her book.

Wendy Cohan has given us a great gift to have researched and written a book linking diet, lifestyle, and genital/urinary tract symptoms. Most people eat foods on a daily basis that do not serve them well. Their choices are not working for them, but without education and awareness, people may continue to suffer without realizing the food they place in their mouths three times a day may be a root cause of their symptoms.

The day-to-day choices of foods that we make for ourselves and our families have profound effects on our health and well-being. For some, their choices serve them well, but for others consuming specific foods can lead to chronic health conditions, pain, and misery. I can speak especially to inflammatory foods and the myriad symptoms and chronic conditions they propel. Inflammatory foods create inflammation in our bodies, which is the basis of most chronic health diseases — from heart disease, diabetes, arthritis, and respiratory and skin disorders to lesser-known conditions that affect every system, including the urinary tract. The role of diet in triggering inflammation cannot be overlooked. Equally, I am adamant about testing for food sensitivities in anyone with a chronic condition, and Wendy elucidates the reasoning for this approach superbly.

All the points that Wendy stresses are keys to vibrant, pain-free heath. Managing stress; getting good sleep, adequate daily hydration, regular exercise, a clean diet; addressing our hormonal balance (both reproductive and adrenal); and assembling a varied medical team of conventional, alternative, and physical medicine providers are your goal points to feeling better in almost any condition, and Wendy presents a compelling case for each of these, in addition to other important, less-intuitive health factors.

I want to especially laud Wendy for teasing out the specific inflammatory element present in some of the most common and dearly loved foods in America: gluten. Gluten is a large, difficult-to-digest protein found in wheat, rye, barley, spelt, and kamut (among other lesser-known grains) and any food or food product made from these grains. Gluten sensitivity is what I call the "great mimicker," because the body's reaction to gluten can disguise itself as any number of symptoms affecting any organ system in the body. I have seen neurological, gynecological, cardiac, urinary, dermatological, musculoskeletal, and other disorders and diseases *vanish* with the complete and diligent elimination of gluten from the diet. Her connection of gluten with interstitial cystitis and other pelvic problems is a point that can't be emphasized and highlighted enough, and the connection is tragically not well disseminated or known in the medical community.

If your doctor won't test for food sensitivities, especially gluten intolerance and celiac disease, search for a doctor who will. Turn over every stone suggested in this book until you feel relief. Assemble a cohesive medical team to support you in every aspect of your healing journey.

If you are a practitioner, may you be enlightened and find answers to help treat your patients and guide them to well-being.

May you find relief if you are suffering from chronic pelvic pain.

— Lisa Shaver, ND, MSOM, LAc
Naturopathic physician, classical Chinese
medicine practitioner, and licensed acupuncturist
Everyday Wellness Clinic, Portland, OR
Faculty National College of Natural Medicine, Portland, OR
Branch Manager of the Portland Metro
Gluten Intolerance Group
www.bewelleveryday.com

Preface

The Better Bladder Book: A Holistic Approach to Healing Interstitial Cystitis and Chronic Pelvic Pain is a comprehensive resource guide and recovery plan covering a complicated subject with clarity, accuracy, and compassion. It examines the most recent peer-reviewed research and is thoroughly documented, but it can also be easily understood by those without a health background. What makes this book relevant is its thesis, which affirms what many women have suspected and research overwhelmingly supports — that interstitial cystitis (IC) is *not* a disease of the bladder alone, but a symptom of underlying dysfunction or imbalance in the body. We have known for well over a decade that IC is associated with other chronic pain syndromes and with autoimmune diseases, yet many practitioners continue to treat IC in isolation and with therapies that are not nearly as effective as patients deserve. We must begin to translate research into action and to transform the way we treat the millions of patients who suffer from IC and other chronic pelvic pain disorders.

This book is my attempt to put into words what I have learned in my own ten-year struggle with IC and chronic pelvic pain. I have personally experienced many of the treatments described in this book. I know that getting well requires a level of commitment strong enough to weather some hills and valleys along the journey. Seldom is anyone's recovery without a few temporary setbacks.

In 1996 I was diagnosed with IC, a painful, chronic, and often-progressive disease. The symptoms mimic those of a severe bladder infection — one that never goes away. Since urine ultimately comes from what we eat and drink, along with waste products from the body's metabolic processes, it made sense to try a dietary approach, even though at the time most doctors gave diet little credit for a reduction in symptoms. I had good luck immediately by excluding known bladder irritants like tomatoes, caffeine, chocolate, citrus, and alcohol. Nevertheless, over the next several years my IC progressed and I eventually needed to take pain medications, antispasmodics, and other medications to enable me to function, especially while working as a hospital RN and raising a family.

After undergoing years of traditional medical treatment, I grew frustrated by the intense focus on symptom management alone and by a failure to investigate other indicators of chronic, systemic illness. No one looked at my body holistically or suggested that any additional symptoms I experienced — mouth ulcers, nutrient malabsorption, fatigue, and more — were of any real concern. Fortunately, I *was* treated with compassion and my pain was taken seriously. I was given medications with which to control my symptoms, but drugs didn't solve all of my bladder problems, and they produced serious side effects.

I made the choice to stop working for a few years to concentrate on rebuilding my health. In my determination to "leave no stone unturned," I began to seek the help of complementary practitioners, experiment with my diet, and undergo testing for food allergies and sensitivities. Careful observation showed me what foods negatively affected my bladder. Eliminating gluten — a protein found in wheat, wheat relatives, barley, rye, and sometimes oats — began to reduce my bladder symptoms and also resolved a chronic skin rash. A conscious effort to reduce stress, deepen my mind–body connection, and manage my daily symptoms with gentle herbal teas rather than prescription medications began to have a very positive effect on my overall health. After about two years of sticking to my routine, plus a lot of complementary body work to further support my system, my bladder gradually healed.

Now, fourteen years after my initial diagnosis, I am pain-free, my urine tests are perfectly normal, and my sleep is no longer interrupted by nighttime voiding. My urologist readily agrees that gluten negatively affects the bladder in some portion of her patients, and that eliminating gluten can lead to a reduction in symptoms. Still, although anecdotal reports abound linking gluten intolerance to bladder problems, there are no published peer-reviewed journal articles on the topic. What is the percentage of IC patients who might be helped by a gluten-free diet? We know this number for other disorders, such as psoriasis (16 percent) and autism (at least 19 percent, and possibly much higher). We need clinical studies to determine the coincidence or comorbidity of IC and other bladder disorders with celiac disease (and with non-celiac gluten sensitivity).

For many years I have advocated a gluten-free diet on IC-support websites. In August of 2008 I published an article on a popular gluten-intolerance website and on my own website (www.gluten freechoice.com), and the response I received was overwhelming. Many people experience gluten-related bladder problems, and I will tell many of their success stories in this book. But it is important to know that gluten isn't the *only* food sensitivity linked to bladder symptoms. Dairy, soy, cane sugar, peanuts, high-oxalate foods, and eggs have also been linked to bladder discomfort, urinary frequency, urinary urgency, and increased incidence of urinary tract infections. Caffeine's negative effect on the bladder is legendary.

This book is all about possibilities. Please believe me when I say that you do not have to live with constant pain or the embarrassment that often comes with chronic pelvic and bladder problems. Anyone who has experienced IC knows that it can mean suffering continuous, disabling pain — pain at the core of our being. This kind of pain affects our psychological and emotional health, our sense of well-being, our self-esteem, and even our sexuality. Please believe that what we eat, how we choose to live, and the way we treat our bodies deeply affect our health. Good luck with your journey to recovery, and know that there are others who can help you along the way.

The best in health.

— Wendy Cohan, RN
Portland, Oregon
www.wellbladder.com
www.glutenfreechoice.com

Acknowledgments

The saying, "Sometimes it takes a village" can apply to matters of health as well as social policy. By "village," I mean my health-care team. Over a decade, this has included many people with the initials MD, ND, PT, DC, LMT, and LNP after their names. I've even, at desperate times, ventured outside of both traditional and naturopathic medicine to speak with energy healers and laypeople with tremendous personal knowledge. Each of us has the capacity to be a healer, a catalyst, a motivator, or a sounding board to those in need of healing. In my journey, several people stand out in their capacity to heal and to listen.

I wish to thank Jaroslava Zoubek, MD, who first diagnosed my IC and has always treated me with compassion and respect. Delinda Free, a highly skilled licensed massage therapist and practitioner of craniosacral therapy, has the hands and heart of a healer, and I am much better off for receiving her care. Joe and Cynthia Keeney, of Keeney Physical Therapy, introduced me to the arts of neurofascial processing, integrative manual therapy, and other adjuncts to traditional physical therapy, and they are directly responsible for speeding my road to recovery. Wendy Larson, PT, taught me about trigger points. B. J. Reid Czarapata, CRNP, CUNP, spoke with me at length regarding infectious disease and IC and offered expert guidance on treatment. Judy Neall, ND, diagnosed and treated my adrenal fatigue and helped balance my hormones.

The initial inspiration for writing this book came from Char Glenn, MD, who also shared her expertise with celiac disease. As I developed *The Better Bladder Book*, others who were invaluable as sounding boards included Lisa Shaver, ND; Leigh Ann Chapman, ND; George Burroughs, DC; Michelle Poirot, LMT; and Kimberly

Skach. Leslie Anderson not only was a sounding board for my ideas, but also read parts of the book, produced the book's figures, and expertly edited my sources. Many thanks to the Boyd family for gracious Montana hospitality and Internet access during the final phase of reviewing the book!

I wish to publicly thank Jeanne Karow and Amrit Willis, RN, for their dedication to helping others with chronic pain and IC on the IC Puzzle support website (see "Resources"), developed by Amrit Willis, which I've been an active contributor to and member of for many years.

There is one more individual to thank: my chief critic, who had the fortune or misfortune to read more about female anatomy and bladder problems than any man should have to, my husband, editor extraordinaire, and all-around support system, David Cohan.

Lastly, I owe a big thank-you to Hunter House Publishers for taking a chance on this book and my talented editors for helping to bring my vision to fruition with a strong dedication to excellence. My deep hope is that this book will change many lives for the better and brighten the future for those with IC and other chronic pelvic pain disorders.

··· Introduction

In this holistic guide to bladder wellness through diet, lifestyle, and self-treatment, you will learn the tools, resources, and practices you need to help you recover your bladder health and alleviate chronic pelvic pain. These tools will continue to be useful as you begin to lead a healthier lifestyle.

The Better Bladder Book is divided into three easy-to-navigate parts, three appendixes, and a guide to resources for further information or support. Those who want to proceed immediately to the recovery portion of the book can skip Part I and move ahead to Part II: "Beginning Your Healing Journey."

Part I, "Finding Your Healing Path," begins with a plea for a new approach to treating chronic pelvic pain disorders and presents clear evidence that interstitial cystitis (IC, a chronic condition of bladder pain and inflammation), in particular, is part of a systemic imbalance that affects many of the body's systems rather than a disease that affects the bladder alone. I discuss the ways in which traditional (allopathic) medicine has been unable to meet the challenges presented by the complexity of IC (also known as painful bladder syndrome [PBS]) and has proven less than successful for far too many patients. I give a brief introduction to the urological system, including anatomical differences between males and females and what happens when things begin to go wrong. I present a clear explanation of common urinary problems, such as stress incontinence, and move on to discuss chronic bladder disorders, such as IC and overactive bladder (OAB), and their associated symptoms. Chapter 3, "Traditional Treatments," is an overview of standard allopathic medical treatments, including medication management and more invasive methods of treatment. Multidisciplinary care by a chronic pain specialty clinic is reviewed, and the first of many success stories is presented.

Part II, "Beginning the Journey," introduces easy-to-learn self-care tools designed to quickly facilitate your recovery. This section is the heart of the book; it is where you learn how to take charge of your own recovery. More success stories have been included to inspire you and to highlight the fact that the path to wellness is unique for each of us.

Part III, "Further Along the Road to Recovery," is for people who say, "I've done everything I can think of, followed all the recommendations I've seen, and I'm still not well." It will guide you in exploring further other health conditions that could be limiting your recovery. You may need to tackle additional challenges, as I have. The additional information on special diets and complementary therapies presented here will assist you in tailoring your recovery plan to your particular needs. This portion of the book concludes with a review of other serious disorders that can potentially cause both pelvic pain and bladder symptoms. This is important information, especially for those with persistent symptoms or an uncertain diagnosis.

The three appendixes include a wealth of information about how to follow the recommended gluten-free diet and also about using medicinal herbs, soothing teas, and homeopathic remedies for bladder symptoms, pelvic pain, and adrenal health, which, as you will learn throughout the book, are intimately intertwined. These are important tools in learning to gain control over the pain and other symptoms you are experiencing.

The Resources section at the back of the book includes a list of helpful books, articles, websites, and organizations involved in research, education, and patient support for people suffering from a variety of pelvic pain disorders.

As you read *The Better Bladder Book*, I hope you will begin to believe that you deserve to be healthy and free of pain, to believe that your bladder can recover, and to believe that once again you'll be able to sleep at night and enjoy your sexuality. Like many important and challenging quests, it sometimes takes a group effort, and the most important person — the one who will need to contribute the greatest effort — is *you*. All you need is a little help.

PART I

Finding
Your Healing Path

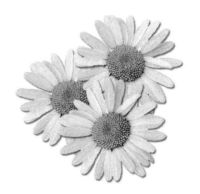

1

A New Approach to Bladder and Pelvic Pain

Bladder and pelvic pain seem to emanate from the core of our beings; it is pain we are not likely to feel comfortable talking about with others. Bladder pain, urinary frequency, and urinary urgency also trigger anxiety. For those of you who *haven't* experienced interstitial cystitis (IC), just think back to a time when you were searching for a shopping mall bathroom or confined to a car while experiencing a full bladder. Those with IC, a painful and debilitating inflammation of the bladder lining and a common source of chronic pelvic pain, often suffer a much more extreme level of discomfort under similar conditions. Now imagine bladder pain that continues, or even worsens, during the night, when the body needs to rest, repair tissue damage, and allow the nervous system to relax. Having IC prevents this repair and restoration from taking place, activating an ongoing cascade of pain and inflammation.

Seeing the Big Picture

IC and chronic pelvic pain can seem very complicated — as if every patient presents a different picture. Rather than making doctors scratch their heads, however, this complexity should suggest that these disorders may have multiple causes, affect many of the body's systems, and are not solely confined to the pelvic area. I believe that physicians who focus on the bladder or prostate *in isolation* are missing the boat, and that this narrow perspective is responsible for the relatively low success rate of existing treatments. Evidence that IC and other pelvic pain disorders are "part of a larger picture" isn't hard to find:

- Many patients with IC or chronic prostatitis (CP) have anecdotally reported that bladder pain increases when eating foods to which they are sensitive; this has now been confirmed in a large study whose results were reported at the 2009 meeting of the American Urological Association. In a survey, 95 percent of female IC patients and 77 percent of male CP patients reported that they had food sensitivities.[1] A Swedish study also reported food sensitivity/allergy as the most frequently encountered comorbid (occurring together) condition among IC patients.[2] And a study of more than 2,400 IC patients found an increased association with allergies.[3]

- Large numbers of those with IC or other forms of chronic pelvic pain reported having additional symptoms or other chronic disorders, including irritable bowel syndrome (IBS), frequent migraines, and vulvodynia (chronic pain around the opening to the vagina).[4] In a recent study involving more than two hundred IC patients, 49 percent reported symptoms that indicated they also had IBS, and 59 percent had symptoms that indicated they had fibromyalgia.[5] In a much larger study, IC patients were one hundred times more likely to suffer from more serious inflammatory bowel disorders, such as Crohn's disease and ulcerative colitis.[6] There is also clinical evidence supporting an association between IC and some autoimmune disorders, such as chronic fatigue syndrome/fibromyalgia, lupus (systemic lupus erythematosus — SLE), and Sjögren's syndrome (see Chapter 2).[7]

These studies and many others help to explain the associated complaints of generalized pain, poor physical quality of life, sleep disturbance, anxiety, depression, fatigue, and feelings of hopelessness commonly reported among those who suffer from chronic pelvic pain in general, and IC in particular.

For patients with IC, the path to healing is shadowed by the knowledge that there is no official cause of or cure for this disorder. Interstitial cystitis affects millions of people in the United States alone, and some patients may suffer through years of misdiagnosis and ineffective treatment before finding appropriate help. IC and other causes of chronic pelvic pain tend to strike those in their thirties and forties — people in the prime of life. They are parents, teachers, businesspeople, and health-care professionals. They are often prominent members of their communities and the primary caregivers and breadwinners for their families.

IC most often coexists with several other sources of chronic pelvic pain, and so I chose to include information on these other conditions in this book. Many of those who suffer from IC and chronic pelvic pain are in constant discomfort, sometimes with little support from family and friends who do not understand these "hidden" disorders that have no outwardly visible symptoms. Only someone who has *experienced* chronic pelvic pain and/or IC can understand the devastating impact of these disorders on a person's life. This is what inspired me to design and implement a holistic recovery plan for IC and other chronic pelvic pain disorders.

New Ways of Thinking about IC and Chronic Pelvic Pain

Why take a holistic approach? Because I believe the standard allopathic approach is "old medicine" and it misses many of the fundamental truths about the underlying causes of interstitial cystitis and chronic pelvic pain. I feel that much more needs to be done by the medical community to diagnose, treat, and ultimately cure IC and related conditions. My personal experience, described below, may help to explain why I truly believe so much more can be done for those with IC and chronic pelvic pain; this experience is echoed by many of the stories shared by others throughout this book.

First, I must state that, with few exceptions, I was treated with compassion and respect by the allopathic medical community and given supportive care and encouragement. Thankfully, my needs for pain medication were addressed. Some people have not been so fortunate. Many people in support groups for IC and chronic bladder pain have related stories of frustration, anger, embarrassment, and disbelief at the way they have been treated by the medical community. (This appears to be changing for the better as more health professionals recognize that IC, overactive bladder, and other chronic pelvic disorders affect a large and growing number of people worldwide.)

Still, I had three major concerns I felt were not thoroughly addressed by the allopathic medical community. First, the role that diet plays in triggering bladder and pelvic inflammation appeared to be largely ignored in clinical practice; specific foods were mentioned only as "irritants." Second, I was very interested in IC and chronic pelvic pain as reflections of systemic and possibly infectious disease, and this, too, seemed to remain unexplored in clinical practice. Finally, a more personal frustration was that no one seemed to be taking a truly holistic approach to chronic pelvic pain. My concerns ultimately led me to devise my own holistic treatment plan, which resulted in my complete recovery from IC. These concerns also played a large role in motivating me to write this book. But the most important reason for developing an alternative treatment plan for IC and chronic pelvic pain is this: The traditional allopathic approach to IC doesn't really work well for many patients. As both a recovered IC patient and a health-care professional, I felt a responsibility to help.

Let's look more closely at these three issues.

The Role of Diet

It occurred to me that since urine ultimately comes from what we eat, maybe what we choose to eat can make a difference in bladder discomfort and other urinary symptoms. When I asked my doctor about this in 1996 I was handed a small dietary pamphlet and was told, "Diet usually doesn't make a difference." Well, it did for me, just as it has for thousands of others, and it can make a big difference for you, too. Within a few weeks on the recommended IC diet, which excludes tomatoes, citrus, vinegar, alcohol, caffeine, and other known bladder irritants, I went into a remission that lasted for several years, with only minor flare-ups when I consumed caffeine. Although this first long remission was not permanent, my disease would certainly have progressed more quickly had I been unable to stay in remission even this long. Diet does help! Just ask anyone who has IC. If there are certain foods that can make symptoms worse, and there almost always are, then avoiding those foods makes good sense. The Interstitial Cystitis Association (ICA) and other organizations strongly support a dietary approach.

I was never tested by my allopathic physicians for food allergies or sensitivities. Later, with the help of complementary-medicine practitioners, I identified my particular food allergies and sensitivities and changed my diet accordingly. Like Jeannie, who shares her story below, doing this has been perhaps the single most important factor in my recovery.

CASE STUDY: *Jeannie's Success Story*

I was diagnosed with severe IC five years ago. I was unable to work for a year and a half and have been on regular pain meds just to get through life. Two weeks ago I went on a salad kick, and a week into it I realized I had no bladder pain or urinary frequency. I thought, "What have I not eaten in a week?" And it dawned on me: bread! What? I love bread! But I was pain-free, and I wasn't foggy-brained or fatigued like I usually am.

I have a friend whose husband has celiac disease, the hereditary form of gluten intolerance. I consulted with him regarding diet and decided to continue the course. I have been gluten-free for almost two weeks. I feel better than I've felt since I was a kid. I ate one English muffin to test my hypothesis and felt like I was going to die the next day. Before going gluten-free, I also had migraines every week, horrible fatigue, severe joint and muscle/back pain, and dizziness.

I'm now sleeping eight hours through the night for the first time in years. I called my urologist's office to tell them, and they seemed to think there would not be a link. I say there most definitely is! It's too bad it took a hysterectomy, removal of my ovaries, and countless other painful and invasive pelvic procedures throughout my life to figure out that gluten intolerance, in the form of celiac disease, was crippling me.

One-Year Update

As of April 2010 I will have been gluten-free for a year. I accidently got "glutened" a couple of weeks ago, and all my symptoms came back. It took a couple of days before I felt back to normal again. Gluten causes my IC to flare up (the most severe consequence I suffer from eating gluten) and also affects my nervous system. When I ingest gluten, I become easily agitated, moody, and tearful (probably from the IC pain), so it's imperative that I stay away from it.

I recently had a yearly physical, and due to some results I had to see a cardiologist. They said I have what is called "Autonomic Nervous System Dysfunction," which causes me to have very low blood pressure, a very low pulse rate, dizziness, fainting, cognitive problems, etc. This disorder goes hand in hand with issues such as fibromyalgia and a huge host of other medical problems. As you know, fibromyalgia is a common problem in people with IC, and many people with IC have multiple health problems. I find this very interesting and personally believe it all goes back to the celiac disease from which I suffer (and which I now know I was born with). Celiac can cause a huge range of problems that can affect both the immune and nervous systems. I understand that doctors want positive proof as to the cause of IC; however, as someone who's dealt with my body more than anyone else, I believe with 200 percent certainty that IC involves a breakdown of the immune system on some level.

I've gone totally organic and preservative-free, and I feel that doing this has helped me tremendously. I still have to follow a gluten-free and IC-friendly diet, but my bladder is not nearly as sensitive as it used to be.

IC and Chronic Pelvic Pain as a Systemic Disease

I have always believed that IC is a systemic disease, regardless of the history of onset or particular symptoms. This possibility wasn't something any of my allopathic physicians appeared to care about. I wasn't routinely tested for markers of inflammation, even though IC is a disease characterized by chronic inflammation. I was never referred to a rheumatologist or a specialist in autoimmune disorders, even though there is evidence linking IC to an autoimmune response. (An autoimmune response occurs when the body's immune system mistakenly attacks the body's cells as "foreign invaders," or enemies, which results in inflammation and tissue destruction.) And

I don't believe that enough of an effort has been made to accurately determine the role of infectious disease in IC and other pelvic inflammatory disorders, although this may be beginning to change.

A Holistic Approach to Treating IC and Chronic Pelvic Pain

I was never referred to a nutritionist, psychologist, endocrinologist, gynecologist, or any other practitioner who could help me figure out why my body was failing me in such a painful and debilitating way. With the exception of sleep patterns, I was never questioned in detail about any other symptoms I might have been experiencing in addition to my bladder symptoms. And it wasn't until after I had a hysterectomy that I learned firsthand the important role hormones play in urogenital health.

IC doesn't affect just the bladder. It deeply affected all of me: my psychological well-being; my sense of self; my roles as wife, mother, nurse, and outdoors enthusiast. IC greatly affected my sexuality, my marriage, my relationships with my children, and more. When my bladder pain was flaring, I didn't feel well *anywhere*. I often felt flushed, as if I had a fever. I had low energy. I felt unwell because I *was* unwell. The bottom line is that no traditional care provider looked at "all of me."

Possible Pathways to IC and Chronic Pelvic Pain

After spending years struggling with IC and reading everything I could get my hands on about the condition, I've come to believe that there are multiple "pathways" to IC and perhaps other chronic pelvic pain disorders. This makes sense for many reasons, but mostly because these conditions are primarily chronic inflammatory disorders, and inflammation can have multiple causes.

Inflammation can result from trauma, from an autoimmune response, or from infection. It can also be driven by the nervous system in a process known as neurogenic inflammation, which we'll discuss in detail in Chapter 7. Inflammation is usually held in check by the hormone cortisol, which is produced by the adrenal glands, but when the demand for increased cortisol never lets up, adrenal fatigue can result, causing reduced energy and an inability to cope with stress. (See Chapter 9 for an in-depth discussion of adrenal fatigue.) When the body is unable to keep up with the demand for cortisol, inflammation begins to get out of hand.

This reasoning leads me to the certainty that the causes of IC — or what I've come to think of as the "triggers" of IC — can include the following:

- **trauma and stress** — acute, and then becoming chronic. Chronic, unrelieved stress can lead to adrenal fatigue, which can result in runaway inflammation. Chronic stress also often leads to an unconscious tightening of the pelvic floor muscles, which in turn can painfully compress the bladder.

- **autoimmune response** — triggered by food allergies or sensitivities, gluten intolerance, celiac disease, leaky gut, gut dysbiosis, or as a result of genetic predisposition. I'll discuss each of these subjects in depth in later chapters, and explain their very real connection with IC.

- **pathogenic organisms** — an occult, or "hidden," infection, caused by Lyme disease, *Bartonella*, *Chlamydia pneumoniae*, *Enterococcus*, or another organism. (Pathogenic organisms are known to cause disease.) Many researchers feel that further research is needed before an infectious cause of IC can be ruled out.

- **occult infection developing secondarily to an existing injury to the bladder lining** — There are various possible causes of injury to the bladder lining, including an ordinary urinary tract infection, an autoimmune inflammatory process triggered by eating gluten (a type of protein found in wheat, barley, and rye), or even neurogenic inflammation (see below) from a musculoskeletal cause. A pathogen may then take advantage of the damaged bladder lining and initiate a process of long-term infection that would otherwise not be possible in a healthy bladder. For example, many women seem to develop IC following a bladder infection that was successfully treated with antibiotics, but their bladders never really feel better. The organism they were being treated for is gone, but another less-easily identified pathogen has invaded the bladder during this vulnerable period.

- **neurogenic inflammation** — inflammation generated by the nervous system, resulting in referred pain from trigger points in response to a variety of factors including pelvic floor dysfunction, spinal disc problems, and postural problems. Neurogenic inflammation may also be related to lifestyle factors such as job routines, too much time spent in a sitting position, or holding urine or stool inappropriately when the body is obviously signaling you to "go."

As the above list indicates, chronic pelvic pain can have several, often-overlapping, triggers. It is possible that IC may be the result of a "perfect storm," with several potential triggers occurring simultaneously. Pull any thread and it has the potential to connect with another: Tissue injury or immune-system compromise can lead to infection, which can lead to inflammation and pain, which can lead to chronic pelvic floor tension, which can lead to neurogenic inflammation, which can lead to increased pain — and so on. Left unchecked, this chain of events can ultimately result in *heightened nervous-system sensitivity and symptoms that are beyond one's ability to control — and sometimes even to cope with*. The scenario described above is reflected in the difficulty of treating IC, and in the fact that many people seem to gain control of their symptoms, and even go into remission, following a variety of treatments, rather than just one type of treatment.

The many factors affecting chronic pelvic pain such as IC can sometimes lead people to make quite passionate posts on support websites. Each person whose health has improved naturally wants to advocate for "their" approach, whether it is a specific diet, physical therapy, or long-term antibiotics. In fact, each of these patients has achieved partial (and often temporary) success by intervening at one of the points on the continuum of pain, inflammation, and heightened nervous-system sensitivity. This is why I believe that the best approach to treating IC and other chronic pelvic pain disorders is to keep turning over stones until you find your solution — or solutions — that will allow you to achieve a complete recovery.

There are many hopeful signs that the tide is turning and that both researchers and clinicians are beginning to view IC holistically. IC researcher and author Dr. Robert Moldwin was recently invited to be a member of a panel on the future of women's health research at the National Institutes of Health (NIH). This meeting was designed to help the NIH develop priorities for research funding in the next few decades. The "Chronic Pain Syndromes" panel that Dr. Moldwin participated in developed some important suggestions to guide future research, perhaps the most significant being to investigate chronic pain syndromes (such as IC) as "systemic" problems — ones affecting multiple bodily systems. Another suggestion was to look at the effect of hormones and diet on chronic pain syndromes.[8] These are very positive and welcome signs for the future of IC treatment. Perhaps medicine is at last beginning to listen to the pleas of millions of patients affected by chronic pelvic pain who have long felt that these conditions are a reflection of a larger systemic problem involving the immune system, the nervous system, and other body systems.

What You Can Do Now

It is extremely important to become an informed consumer of health care so you can help direct your own healing journey. For example, if you have a family history of celiac disease and you develop IC, then testing for food sensitivities, especially gluten intolerance, is an obvious place to start. If you suffered birth trauma during the delivery of your child and shortly afterward began having bladder issues or discomfort with intercourse, then undergoing a thorough evaluation by a physical therapist trained in pelvic floor rehabilitation would be one of the first things to do. If you have other health problems in addition to IC-like symptoms and fatigue, and you live in an area where deer ticks carry Lyme disease, then perhaps testing for Lyme, as well as its associated pathogens, may be your priority. We will discuss all of these areas of treatment throughout this book; meanwhile, keep turning over those stones!

IC and chronic pelvic pain are both persistent health problems. They place an unrelieved burden on our adrenal glands and our stress-response system. We know that the adrenal glands, which control our fight-or-flight response, are adversely affected by chronic stress. Stress, both chronic and acute, comes in many forms — physical, psychological, and emotional. And anyone with IC or another form of chronic pelvic pain is likely to suffer from all of these forms of stress. You'll learn more about this critical link between chronic pain, the nervous system, and bladder health throughout *The Better Bladder Book*. Let's stop the cycle of pain and support our bodies to heal.

2

Understanding the Basics

Learning a little about how the urinary system functions makes it easier to understand what happens when things don't work the way they should. This chapter describes the anatomy and physiology of the female and male urinary systems, and discusses the basic types of urinary dysfunction, before focusing more closely on interstitial cystitis (IC) and chronic pelvic pain.

Understanding the Urinary System

Normally, the urinary system is composed of two kidneys, two ureters (the tubes that carry urine from the kidney to the bladder), the bladder, and the urethra (the tube that leads from the bladder to the external opening). There are also several important rings of muscle called sphincters, which can constrict or relax as needed to prevent or allow the flow of urine. The body is very adaptable and can do well with only one healthy, functioning kidney. This is why close relatives and even properly matched anonymous donors can give one of their kidneys to someone with kidney disease who would otherwise have to stay on dialysis for the rest of their life. Less commonly, someone is born with only one kidney; as long as they stay healthy, they can live a normal life.

Our bodies discharge waste products through the lungs, skin, intestines, and bladder. These waste products come from what we eat and from our metabolic functions. When the proteins we eat are broken down, our kidneys remove a waste product called urea from the blood and pass it through an incredibly efficient filtration system to be excreted from the body. Urine is made up of urea, water, toxins, and excesses of other substances the body doesn't need. From the kidneys, urine travels down the ureters into the bladder in small increments several times a minute; we normally feel the urge to urinate when the bladder's "collection container" is nearing capacity.

In both genders, the bladder is a hollow organ located within the pelvis. It consists primarily of smooth muscle protected on the interior surface by two stretchy layers of tissue called mucosa, similar to the moist, flexible tissue that lines the intestines. These mucosal layers are critical in maintaining a comfortable bladder. When healthy and intact, they serve to prevent injury to the underlying muscle layer from the acids, salts, and toxins contained in urine.

The bladder's innermost mucosal layer, sometimes referred to as the glycosaminoglycan (GAG) layer, is made up of GAGs and glycoproteins. The GAG layer plays a protective role, preventing harm to the epithelial cells that lie beneath. It is able to do this because it is hydrophilic or "water-loving" — it contains an ionic charge that holds a layer of water between the epithelium and the bladder contents.[1] This layer of water plays a dual purpose: It helps to repel harmful organisms and prevent urinary tract infection, and it protects the bladder epithelium from injury.[2] This remarkable system usually works very well. However, people with IC usually have a defective GAG layer, which lets the irritating salts, acids, and toxins through the protective barrier to the sensitive tissues beneath, causing the pain, sensitivity, urinary frequency, and urinary urgency of IC.

The outside of the bladder is encased in and supported by a layer of connective tissue called fascia. Fascia can sometimes become restricted, limiting movement and triggering discomfort and spasticity. This frequently happens as a result of scar tissue formation.

The urethra, a much shorter tube than the ureters, leads from the bottom "neck" of the bladder to the external opening known as the urethral orifice. The urethra contains special glands that secrete protective mucous into the urethral canal. This mucous is important in helping to prevent irritation in the urethra from the passage of urine.

The Female Urological System

In females the urethra is fairly short, about four centimeters (or slightly less than two inches) (see Figure 2.1). This makes it relatively easy for fecal bacteria to enter and migrate up the urinary tract to cause infection in the bladder. The urethral orifice (external opening) is located within the vulva, just above the vaginal opening. The urethra in females is designed to carry only urine and mucous secretions. At the point where the bladder empties into the urethra (bladder neck) lies an internal urethral sphincter, a ring of muscular tissue that helps to prevent involuntary leakage of urine (stress incontinence). There is also an external urethral sphincter, called the urogenital diaphragm.

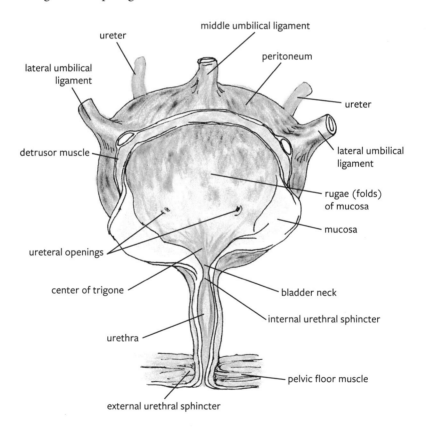

FIGURE 2.1 Female bladder anatomy

The Male Urological System

In males, the urethra is much longer than in females, and it is made up of three distinct parts (see Figure 2.2).

Males have a donut-shaped organ called the prostate gland surrounding the urethra. The "prostatic" section of the urethra must pass through this walnut-sized gland, which can cause problems later in life as the prostate gland enlarges, sometimes constricting the flow of urine. This can be a serious problem for older men, resulting in the need to void small amounts frequently, interrupting sleep and the activities of daily life and increasing the risk of urinary tract infection.

The "membranous" section of the male urethra passes through the urogenital diaphragm.

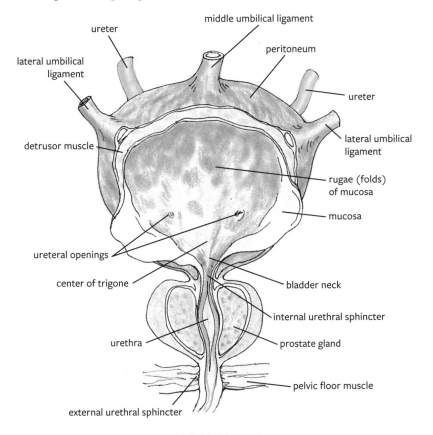

FIGURE 2.2 Male bladder anatomy

The final, or "spongy," section of the male urethra passes through the penis to the urethral meatus, or external orifice. In males, both urine and seminal fluid from the reproductive organs pass through the urethra. This requires great elasticity to accommodate a larger flow during both urination and sexual activity.

Urination

When things are working the way they're supposed to, the system of urinary elimination follows a predictable pattern. Initially the person feels a slight need to urinate, which increases in intensity as the bladder approaches capacity. The powerful detrusor muscle (part of the bladder wall), the perineal muscles (at the bottom of the pelvic floor), the muscles of the abdominal wall, the muscles of the urethral sphincters, and even the thoracic diaphragm (located beneath the lungs) are all involved in the process of building pressure within the bladder. These muscles relax once the nerves have succeeded in transmitting the urge to empty the bladder. When we urinate, the nerves and accessory muscles work together to simultaneously contract the bladder muscle and relax the sphincter muscle. These two events need to happen in the right order to provide a normal pattern of urination.

Lots of important things happen in the pelvis; it is no wonder that the bladder and surrounding organs contain a large number of nerves. Along with signaling other powerful sensations, of course, they tell us when it is time to empty the bladder. Hyperexcitability of these nerves is thought to be a factor in the development of overactive bladder, interstitial cystitis, and other sources of chronic pelvic pain. An overstimulated nervous system is also associated with tissue inflammation, one of the cardinal signs of not only IC, but also of many other chronic diseases.[3]

Urinary Dysfunction: What's Happening with My Body?

So that's how things are supposed to work. What happens when they don't? Unfortunately, this is an ever-present and distressing problem for the more than 15 million Americans who suffer from chronic urinary symptoms.[4] However, since not everyone suffers from IC, we'll begin with some information on the common causes of bladder symptoms and offer possible solutions. Then, in the next section, we'll begin an in-depth discussion of IC and chronic pelvic pain, which are the main topics of this book. I've also included a section on urinary tract problems in men. And in an effort to leave no stone unturned, I've included in Chapter 11 important information on other potentially serious conditions that can cause urinary symptoms.

Urinary Tract Infection

By far the most common problem causing bladder symptoms is a urinary tract infection (UTI). For this reason, it is very important to rule out active infection before attempting any self-treatment plan for bladder problems. Pay a visit to your physician and ask for a urine culture. Urinary tract infections can become kidney infections, which are extremely painful. Any infection can result in sepsis (a serious medical condition involving a whole-body or "systemic" inflammatory response triggered by infection) and become life-threatening.

The symptoms of a UTI are caused by the body's inflammatory response to invasion by pathogenic microorganisms. (A UTI is referred to as a bladder infection or cystitis if it affects the lower urinary tract, that is, the urethra and bladder.) UTI is the most frequently encountered bacterial infection, accounting for seven million visits to doctors annually in the United States alone. UTIs are responsible for a million emergency room visits annually, resulting in a hundred thousand hospital admissions. The total cost of treating non-hospital-acquired UTIs in the United States is estimated to be more than 1.6 billion dollars (2002 figures).[5]

For various reasons, including their anatomy, women are at a greater risk than men, and nearly half of all women will experience at least one UTI in their lifetime.[6] Normal sexual activity increases the likelihood of contracting a UTI. In people under age fifty, UTI is far less common in men than in women and is usually associated with some other type of urological abnormality. However, in older men, as mentioned, benign enlargement of the prostate gland can result in obstructed flow of urine and increase the risk of UTI.

Certain groups of people, including both older men and older women, are at greater risk of developing UTI, although symptoms may not easily be recognized, and some infections may be completely asymptomatic. Reasons for the increase in risk with aging may include a general decrease in immunity, an increase in fecal and urinary incontinence, and an increase in neurologic and cognitive dysfunction. Another factor can be increased exposure to health-care-associated infections (HAIs), which sometimes result from hospitalization and institutionalization in long-term-care centers.[7]

Other populations that face an increased risk of both UTI and complications from UTI include those with diabetes, HIV, multiple sclerosis, spinal cord injury, and those who are pregnant.[8]

At least 80 percent of UTIs are caused by *Escherichia coli* (*E. coli*). *Staphylococcus* species account for another 10–15 percent of infections. The remaining cases usually result from other bacteria, including *Klebsiella* spp., *Proteus mirabilis*, and *Enterococcus faecalis*. In women especially, the sexually transmitted microorganism *Chlamydia trachomatis* may infect the urinary tract. More complicated cases of UTI can involve the microorganisms *Serratia marcescens*, *Pseudomonas aeruginosa*, group B *Streptococci*, and *Candida albicans* (a fungus, not a bacterium).

⁕ Prevention

Two pieces of advice we often hear for preventing or treating bladder infections are to increase overall liquid intake and to drink cranberry juice. Although increasing liquid intake may indeed help to flush bacteria from the urinary tract and prevent infections from developing, it also dilutes our natural immune defenses.[9] And in people who have partial obstruction of the urethra from an enlarged prostate or other causes, forcing fluids can result in urine retention and actually lead to a UTI. The best advice may be to follow these simple principles: Drink when you're thirsty; drink enough to maintain clear, light-yellow urine; and always increase liquid intake when you have a fever.

Cranberry juice has been favored for the prevention of urinary tract infection because it was thought to increase the acidity of the urine, thereby creating an environment that does not favor bacterial growth. Several earlier studies did not support this theory. Recent studies, however, have identified the cranberry components fructose and proanthocyanidins as having the potential to prevent bacterial adherence to epithelial cells in the urinary tract and bladder, thus decreasing the chances of developing an infection.[10] This factor may be especially important in the case of *E. coli*, the most common urinary pathogen. But, overall, the recommendation for consumption of cranberry juice for prevention or treatment of UTI requires additional long-term and larger studies. It should also be noted that those with IC are often unable to tolerate drinking cranberry juice, at least until their bladder lining has begun to heal, as it worsens pain.

Hygiene is sometimes overlooked as a major strategy in the prevention of UTI. We've all heard the old adage about wiping from front to back, and it is still great advice. It is especially important if you suffer occasionally or frequently from loose stools. Regular, frequent showering is important, always using the front-to-back cleansing strategy. It may seem like a good idea to use vaginal cleansing products or douches, but they aren't necessary, and they have the potential to disrupt normal, healthy vaginal bacterial flora. One of the most important hygiene practices you can implement is for you and your partner to wash before *and* after engaging in sex. Ideally, this should include the mouth, the genitals, and any other areas where intimate contact is likely to occur.

Another possible cause of bladder infection is irregular voiding, or holding urine for too long, which allows any bacteria present to adhere to the bladder lining and begin to multiply, rather than being flushed out at regular intervals. Doctors sometimes see a spike in UTIs during ski season, when long lines and bulky clothing make a trip to the restroom impractical. (The guys usually take care of this in the out-of-bounds area.) A long car ride with no bathroom access may produce the same result. It is important to drink water regularly and to void regularly; this is how our bodies are designed to function properly.

❋ Symptoms

So, if prevention didn't work, and you begin to feel some of the following symptoms, you may have developed a UTI. Symptoms involving the lower urinary tract can include discomfort with urination; cloudy urine (which may contain a large number of white blood cells, blood, or mucus); urinary frequency or urgency; a sensation of tenderness, heaviness, or abnormal warmth just above the pubic bone; and a peculiar odor and/or color to the urine.

In addition to these symptoms, infection that has progressed up the ureters to involve the upper urinary tract and kidneys involves fever and pain in the flank or mid-back, which may be only one-sided. This type of infection is known as pyelonephritis, and symptoms may progress to a feeling of extreme weakness, severe nausea and vomiting, and unremitting pain. Left untreated, pyelonephritis is *life-threatening*. Pyelonephritis during pregnancy can cause complications, including premature labor. If you suspect you may have this condition, seek treatment immediately!

☀ *Diagnosis*

Because UTI is a common infection, diagnosis is very routine. The patient with symptoms of UTI is asked to give a "clean-catch" urine specimen, which is then dipped with a special stick that tests a number of parameters, such as levels of glucose, blood, leukocytes (white blood cells), pH, and ketones (formed when the body breaks down fat). A high number of white blood cells indicates infection. Next, the urine is checked for the presence of infection and cultured for bacterial growth. Because new strains of antibiotic-resistant organisms are emerging, it is also very important for the laboratory to test the urine culture with a range of possible antibiotics to determine which kills the largest number of organisms in a given time period before the lab recommends an appropriate antibiotic treatment to the physician. Together these processes are known as a "culture and sensitivity" test.

☀ *Treatment*

In the past, doctors frequently prescribed the use of prescription or over-the-counter Pyridium (phenazopyridine hydrochloride), a common bladder analgesic, but this medication has not been shown to be very effective in clinical trials. The drug, which is also found in over-the-counter remedies, frequently causes headaches, rashes, and gastrointestinal discomfort, and it can occasionally have serious adverse reactions such as acute kidney failure and hemolytic anemia. The Canadian Pharmacy Association states that phenazopyridine hydrochloride is not recommended for treatment of routine UTI, especially because symptoms normally resolve quickly after beginning antibiotic treatment.[11]

Rest may be important to recovery, along with easy access to a bathroom so that voiding can take place as often as needed. This is important since urinary frequency and urgency are common symptoms, and holding in urine will only aggravate discomfort.

The treatment of choice for UTI is prescription antibiotics. Although there are herbal antimicrobials that have the potential to help alleviate UTI, given the severe consequences if infection is left unchecked, traditional Western medicine is the *best* choice for a diagnosed UTI. Alternative methods are best left in the "prevention" category, discussed above.

Some commonly used antibiotics include trimethoprim with sulfamethoxazole (Bactrim), which can rarely cause serious hypersensitivity reactions, and quinolones (Levaquin, Cipro), which should not be used when treating children, as there is no established record of safety or effectiveness. Another drug of choice may be nitrofurantoin (Macrobid or Macrodantin), which has the potential to cause serious reactions with long-term use. Doxycycline is effective against a wide range of bacteria, including spirochetes (such as *Borrelia*), which are a group of bacteria whose unique characteristics make them harder to detect and treat. Occasionally, a UTI involves fungal organisms such as *Candida albicans*, and then an antifungal medication, such as fluconazole (or less commonly amphotericin B), is prescribed.[12]

If the symptoms of your UTI persist even after your doctor says the infection is gone, you may want to ask him or her about testing you for IC, which can feel like a bladder infection that just never entirely goes away, or in some cases even worsens.

Overactive Bladder

Overactive bladder, or OAB, is a term used to describe a condition in which urinary frequency and urgency interfere with normal patterns of daily living. OAB is thought to be extremely common; certainly the large number of television ads for OAB treatments has increased our general awareness of the problem.

❊ Symptoms

The primary symptom of OAB is bladder contractions that trigger the urge to void even without a full bladder. Urgency and incontinence often occur together, and being forced to hold urine can lead to incontinence. OAB can also exist as a symptom of IC. But one of the key differences between IC and OAB is nighttime frequency. Unlike their IC counterparts, patients with OAB generally do not get up in excess of four times per night. Pain may or may not be a part of the symptoms experienced with OAB, but it *is* usually a symptom of IC. With OAB, though, pain is usually less common.

❊ Diagnosis

OAB is usually diagnosed based on symptoms described by the patient, sometimes in conjunction with tests to eliminate other possibilities. Don't automatically accept that your OAB is a permanent part of your life. One possibility to consider is that overactive bladder may be caused by an undiagnosed food sensitivity, such as gluten intolerance, that is causing irritation in the bladder or urethra, which in turn triggers the urge to void. Coffee is another good example of a potentially irritating substance, and it is one that we often consume in large quantities. In fact, many women I know admit that they experience more of the spasms that trigger the urge to void when they're drinking more coffee than usual. Maybe there are things you can do to nip your urgency and frequency in the bud before it becomes a serious problem.

❊ Treatment

Overactive bladder can be treated, but if ongoing incontinence is a problem for you, make use of absorbent pads such as Poise brand pads, which are made for this purpose.

Stress reduction, behavioral changes, bladder retraining, and "scheduled voiding" may be very helpful in managing overactive bladder. Some patients have had success with pelvic floor exercises or pelvic floor rehabilitation under the direction of a physical therapist specializing in the treatment of pelvic disorders. There are numerous medications, such as Detrol (tolterodine), Ditropan, Vesicare, and Enablex, available to help control symptoms of OAB. Be aware that constipation and dry mouth are common side effects of this class of medications. Moreover, some studies comparing medication use with the complementary treatment strategies described above suggest that these types of behavioral changes can reduce overactive bladder symptoms with far fewer side effects.

Bladder retraining is aimed at increasing bladder capacity and normalizing voiding patterns by gradually increasing the time between voids, regulating fluid intake, and learning relaxation techniques to avoid the sense of extreme urgency. Although proven helpful in cases of overactive bladder, bladder retraining alone will not help to treat frequency in IC if pain is involved, and having pain is one of IC's chief characteristics. Suppressing the urge to void when pain is present may trigger nervous system symptoms such as profuse sweating, hot flashes, and irritability. Rather than alleviating symptoms, forcibly holding urine during pain, spasms, and other symptoms of IC seems to heighten nervous system responses and increase pain. When at all possible, void as soon as the urge is felt. Sipping water throughout the day, and drinking fewer irritating fluids such as soda, tea, and coffee, is one way to naturally increase your bladder capacity.

As the inflammation and pain of IC are brought under control, bladder capacity and the length of time between voids will naturally increase, unless the damage to the bladder and the development of scar tissue prevents this degree of normalization and healing from occurring.

Stress Incontinence

Stress incontinence is a medical term that refers to the accidental leakage of urine under physically "stressful" situations. This means leaking urine when you cough, sneeze, laugh, drive over large speed bumps, jump rope, run, bend over to tie your shoes, or do the downward dog yoga pose — not necessarily when you have a spat with your husband or your taxes are overdue.

·⁕· Diagnosis

To obtain an accurate diagnosis, and to learn what factors may be causing stress incontinence, you will need to see a gynecologist, a urologist, or a physician with training in both areas — a urogynecologist. The doctor may ask you to perform several maneuvers and to place yourself in different positions to help her or him determine if anatomical changes may be contributing to your condition. Stress incontinence is often attributed to a dropped or fallen bladder, which we'll discuss next, and sometimes additionally to hormonal changes.

·⁕· Treatment

Stress incontinence, too, may be able to be treated. For some women, bladder retraining, which is discussed above, may be helpful. Continued dribbling or wetness can lead to soreness of the vaginal tissues surrounding the urethral opening. This is especially true if you suffer from vaginal dryness or vulvodynia. You may find that in addition to wearing a pad, using a barrier cream, such as the original Eucerin-brand cream, may prevent discomfort from developing. Avoid using ointments that contain zinc oxide, which can be drying. Another tip is to avoid some specific relaxing herbs, such as chamomile, which can actually *increase* incontinence and dribbling. While an excellent herb for the bladder, chamomile is best used for urinary hesitancy, spasms, and pelvic floor dysfunction, *not* incontinence.

Inflammation can play a very big role in creating the conditions that produce stress incontinence. This is only one of several reasons why younger women may experience stress incontinence, even though many people associate this disorder with aging. You may find that following an anti-inflammatory diet, avoiding your specific food allergens, getting the correct balance of essential fatty acids, and getting moderate exercise will dramatically reduce your stress incontinence. I believe that the role of inflammation in stress incontinence is often overlooked.

From a personal perspective, I've gone from experiencing daily stress incontinence to running, hiking, and chasing dogs and Frisbees without needing to wear a pad, simply by gaining control over pelvic inflammation. How could this be? Excess fluid in the confined space of the pelvic cavity presses on the relatively small bladder, which relieves some of that pressure by releasing urine through the urethra. In this light, stress incontinence makes perfect sense — and so does the solution. If you eliminate the excess fluid caused by pelvic inflammation, stress incontinence has a chance to improve. This is a somewhat simplistic perspective, and there are other anatomical conditions that contribute to stress incontinence. A really skilled physical therapist may be a huge help in your individual situation.

Kegel exercises are recommended for women who have problems with incontinence due to weakened muscles related to age or childbirth; a physical therapist can assess your muscle strength and help you develop a strengthening program with specific exercises tailored to your body. You can experiment with locating the correct pelvic floor muscles by trying to stop and start the flow of urine, and by squeezing around your partner's penis or finger during sexual activity. Squeeze gently and rhythmically, and relax completely between each contraction. In addition to helping control stress incontinence, strengthening these pelvic muscles may result in a more satisfying sexual experience over time.[13] Start slowly, and gradually increase the number of repetitions.

Kegel exercises, done correctly, improve blood flow to the pelvic area and strengthen the specific muscles that support the pelvic floor. Studies have shown that three-quarters of women who do Kegel exercises correctly can overcome their stress incontinence.[14]

If doing Kegel exercises causes you any pain, *stop*. Pain during these exercises is not normal. Discuss your findings with a physical therapist who specializes in women's health issues.

Cystocele (Dropped, or Fallen, Bladder)

A cystocele is a condition in which the internal musculature that suspends and supports the bladder fails, and the bladder prolapses, or drops, at least partially into the vagina. It occurs when the wall separating the bladder from the vagina is weakened or thinned by anatomical changes that take place during pregnancies and births, or due to drastic weight loss. It is often exacerbated by repetitive heavy lifting, straining to have bowel movements, or age-related physical changes, including declining estrogen. Estrogen (along with testosterone) is helpful in maintaining normal tissue and muscle tone in the vaginal walls.[15]

✳ Symptoms

Symptoms can include a feeling of fullness in the vagina, urinary frequency, discomfort walking, and stress incontinence, especially when a woman coughs, sneezes, laughs, or performs certain yoga positions, such as downward dog.

✳ Diagnosis

You'll need to see your gynecologist for an accurate diagnosis and to develop a treatment plan, if necessary. A cystocele can occur in varying degrees. A mild, grade-1 cystocele is present if the bladder drops a short distance into the vagina, even intermittently. In a grade-2 cystocele, the bladder may drop low into the vagina, near the opening.

✳ Treatment

For a mild cystocele, physical therapy to strengthen the surrounding muscles is often successful and can help patients avoid eventual surgery. Kegel exercises and other exercises are certainly a good place to start. Some physicians may recommend a pessary, a diaphragm-like device placed inside the vagina to help hold the bladder in place. These come in a variety of sizes and shapes to fit different anatomies. You need to be evaluated by both a gynecologist and a urologist, or by a urogynecologist. For an excellent and compassionate source of information and treatment for pelvic prolapse, stress incontinence, and musculoskeletal sources of pelvic pain, read *Heal Pelvic Pain: A Proven Stretching, Strengthening, and Nutrition Program for Relieving Pain, Incontinence, IBS, and Other Symptoms Without Surgery,* by Amy Stein, MPT.

A grade-3, or advanced, cystocele occurs when the bladder prolapses completely, or protrudes, through the vaginal opening. Unless the patient is opposed (perhaps due to religious beliefs), a grade-3 cystocele usually requires surgical intervention. After evaluation, your surgeon may suggest a bladder suspension or "bladder lift." In a common procedure, the surgeon makes an incision in the upper wall of the vagina to repair and secure the tissues that help to support the bladder. Although there is not usually a long recovery from this procedure, it does involve a short hospital stay, and patients are prohibited from lifting or other straining activities until fully healed, which usually takes about six to eight weeks.

Rectocele, which is a related condition, is a protrusion of the rectum through the vaginal opening, and it is also caused by a weakening of the surrounding muscles. Some women can have both a cystocele and a rectocele.

Nocturia

Nocturia is the medical term for nighttime voiding. People with IC, OAB, or prostate problems may need to void multiple times per night. Your physician may ask you the number of times you get up each night to void, or ask you to keep a "voiding diary." Nocturia can also be caused by taking diuretic medications for heart failure or high blood pressure, or by drinking or eating beverages and foods that have a diuretic effect. These include many herbal teas, culinary herbs like parsley, vegetables like asparagus, and fruits like watermelon. Eating a meal of tabouli salad, made with lots of parsley, with a side of asparagus and a dessert of watermelon will almost guarantee a potent diuretic effect. Add some herbal tea at bedtime and you'll be up all night! In fact, eating asparagus is a folk remedy for congestive heart failure or fluid retention. Watch your fluid intake, too, especially after the dinner hour. This is especially important for children with bed-wetting issues or who are waking several times at night (and waking their parents) to use the bathroom.

FAQs | Urinary Dysfunction

Q: *What could cause bed-wetting in an older child?*
A: One possibility is undiagnosed food sensitivies or allergies. A pediatric allergist or naturopath can test for allergies and food sensitivities and help develop a modified diet for your child. Your pediatrician should already have ruled out any anatomical/structural reasons for your child's bed-wetting. In some cases, this problem can be cleared up very quickly following the elimination of specific foods.

For more information, please refer to the article "Genito-Urinary Problems in Children and Food Allergy" at www.nutramed.com

/children/children_bladder_kidneys.htm (5/2/2009). (Also see the Resources section at the back of the book for further information on dealing with children's urinary issues.)

Q: *Is voiding frequently a normal part of pregnancy, or is something wrong?*

A: Hormonal changes can trigger frequent voiding in the first trimester, and the weight of the fetus resting on the bladder can trigger frequent voiding in the last trimester. If you continue to experience frequent voiding throughout the *second* trimester, mention your concerns to your ob-gyn or nurse-midwife and make sure that she or he has given you the standard test for gestational diabetes, another possible cause of urinary frequency during pregnancy. Due to hormonal changes, some pregnant women may develop urinary tract infections, which would increase urinary frequency but would most likely also trigger additional symptoms such as burning and discomfort with urination.

Of course, urinary frequency may be a symptom of IC. IC in pregnancy has not been well studied, but researchers believe that it does not adversely affect fertility or fetal health. Some women find that their IC goes into remission during pregnancy, while others experience a worsening of their symptoms.[16] It may help to seek the support of another woman who has gone through pregnancy with IC. Online support groups can be very helpful in offering other patients' personal perspectives, but use caution when considering any medical advice given in these forums. Always check with your health practitioner before proceeding with treatment.

Q: *Can I pass my bladder disorder to my sexual partner?*

A: With regard to ordinary UTI, most medical sources say "no." Cases of UTI in women can occur after frequent sexual intercourse (sometimes called "honeymoon cystitis") because during sex, bacteria from the vagina can be pushed through the urethral opening into the urinary tract. (Ordinary UTI is less common in younger and middle-aged men than it is in women in these age groups.) On the other hand, chronic, persistent, and occult bacterial infections (that is, "hidden" infections that impart no symptoms) present more of a gray area. There is some anecdotal evidence that transmission *can* occur between sexual partners, especially when one partner harbors an occult infection, and sexual contact is frequent and ongoing.

(cont'd.)

In persistent cases of contagious chronic illness, it is a good practice to look at all possible sources of transmission, including sexual
partners. This is even true of strep throat, as some people may
be asymptomatic carriers of *streptococcus* bacteria in their nasal
passages.

Chronic Pelvic Pain and Interstitial Cystitis

Although women represent the majority of patients diagnosed with
some form of chronic pelvic pain, men also suffer pelvic pain disorders, including chronic prostatitis (CP), pelvic floor dysfunction,
and IC, all of which we'll learn more about throughout the book. My
hope is that both men and women with these painful disorders benefit from this book and that it provides the necessary information to
enable readers to engage in a proactive discussion with their physicians.

Table 2.1 lists many of the sources of pelvic pain. Some affect only
women, some affect both sexes, and some affect only men. These lists
contain some specific medical terms, which are discussed throughout the book.

Defining Chronic Pelvic Pain (CPP)

It can be quite daunting trying to understand the many names and
definitions associated with CPP. Simply put, chronic pelvic pain is
any pattern of pain affecting the pelvic region of the body that is
ongoing or "chronic" in nature (usually lasting longer than three
months in duration). Some of the uncertainty regarding the definitions of CPP stems from the tendency for all medical practitioners —
not just doctors — to define conditions in terms of their own fields of
specialization. For example, physical therapists write about, conduct
research on, and treat chronic pelvic pain, too, and have their own
terminology and language.

Here are some further clarifications:

- CPP can affect both women and men. In men, it may more often be referred to as chronic pelvic pain syndrome, or CPPS. In
  women, the term "chronic pelvic pain" is often used to describe
  gynecological disorders.

TABLE 2.1: Sources of Chronic Pelvic Pain and Bladder Symptoms

WOMEN ONLY	Endometriosis, including bladder endometriosis
	Ovarian cancer
	Vulvodynia and vulvar vestibulitis
	Urethral syndrome
BOTH WOMEN AND MEN	Chronic urinary tract infection
	IBS-related sacral nerve cross-reactivity/referred pain
	IC/painful bladder syndrome or urgency-frequency-pain syndrome
	Musculoskeletal dysfunction
	Lumbar and sacral disc problems
	Piriformis syndrome
	Iliopsoas syndrome
	Neurological disorders (e.g., multiple sclerosis, normal pressure hydrocephalus)
	Pelvic adhesions from abdominal surgeries
	Pelvic congestion
	Pelvic floor dysfunction (PFD)/tension myalgia of the pelvic floor
	Pudendal neuralgia or pudendal nerve compression syndrome
MEN ONLY	Acute bacterial prostatitis
	Chronic bacterial prostatitis
	Chronic nonbacterial prostatitis, including the alternate names chronic pelvic pain syndrome (CPPS), prostatodynia, pelvic myoneuropathy

- CPP can cause symptoms that are both recurring/intermittent and chronic. The pain may be localized or diffuse.
- Periods of exacerbation and remission are common.
- CPP can cause intermittent or continuous urinary symptoms.
- CPP can cause sexual dysfunction in both men and women.
- CPP can cause significant stress in the lives of patients, their partners, and their family members.
- CPP can develop from a variety of causes; there is rarely a single cause (see Table 2.2 on the next page). In fact, chronic pelvic pain usually has several, often interrelated, causes. To further

illustrate this point, Table 2.2 represents four different patterns
of pain in hypothetical patients suffering from a variety of causes
of pelvic disorders. Patients A through D are not real patients,
but their collections of symptoms represent actual combinations that have been known to occur. The table is intended to
illustrate how common it is to suffer from *three or more* associated and interrelated causes of CPP, perhaps because one factor
often can lead to the development of another. Again, the medical
terms used here are discussed in this chapter and elsewhere in
the book.

TABLE 2.2: Patterns of Chronic Pelvic Pain

FACTORS CONTRIBUTING TO CPP	PATIENT A (FEMALE)	PATIENT B (FEMALE)	PATIENT C (FEMALE)	PATIENT D (MALE)
Piriformis syndrome				✔
Chronic nonbacterial prostatitis				✔
Interstitial cystitis	✔		✔	✔
Pelvic floor dysfunction			✔	
Endometriosis	✔		✔	
Pelvic congestion	✔			
Pelvic adhesions	✔			
Urethral syndrome		✔		
Chronic UTI		✔		
Vulvodynia		✔	✔	

Interstitial Cystitis (IC)

IC is a painful condition characterized by chronic inflammation of
the bladder lining, and it involves aspects of the immune, endocrine,
and nervous systems.[17] As shown in Table 2.2, IC can and often does
exist along with other causes of chronic pelvic pain, as well as with
a variety of autoimmune disorders. IC is often underdiagnosed or
misdiagnosed due to the variability in symptoms. IC is also called

painful bladder syndrome (PBS) and is often referred to as IC/PBS in the medical literature. In Europe it has recently undergone a name change — the new official designation is bladder pain syndrome (BPS) — and in some Asian countries IC is known as hypersensitive bladder syndrome (HBS). For the sake of simplicity, throughout the remainder of the book I will use the term IC exclusively.

Until recently, most researchers and medical practitioners agreed that IC had no known cause (or etiology). Many questions remain to be answered regarding this painful and sometimes disabling disorder. Is IC a problem of nervous system hyperexcitability, or central nervous system "upregulation"? Is it a biological defect or abnormality in the bladder lining? Is it an autoimmune disorder, or an allergic response? IC exhibits *all* of these elements, which we'll discuss throughout the book. The difficulty may lie in sorting out cause and effect. One thing we do know is that IC is *much* more common than we believed just a few years ago.

A large epidemiological study, called the Rand Interstitial Cystitis Epidemiology (RICE) study, was conducted in nearly 100,000 households across the United States.[18] Based on detailed interview questions developed cooperatively by eight IC researchers, the results were analyzed and interpreted to estimate the frequency of IC. Previously, IC has been estimated to affect between 750,000 and 900,000 people in the United States, about 90 percent of whom were women.[19] In contrast, the RICE study, published in 2009, found that 3 to 6 percent of women over age eighteen met the diagnostic criteria for IC.[20] That means *over four million U.S. women* may have IC, and, the disorder is often misdiagnosed in men, who may actually have IC with greater frequency than previously estimated.[21] A small number of children may also be affected.

❊ Symptoms

IC is characterized by symptoms of urinary frequency and urgency, usually accompanied by pain. Sometimes the term "irritative voiding" is used to describe these types of symptoms. IC is often progressive, with symptoms worsening over time, especially when effective treatment is not obtained. It is characterized by periods when symptoms abruptly worsen, called "flares," and periods when symptoms seem to disappear, called "remissions." Flares can last from days to weeks, and remissions can last from weeks to months, or even years in some cases. This is one of several aspects of IC that are similar to those of an autoimmune disease.

Discomfort is partially relieved by emptying the bladder, and it is worsened by having a full bladder. Patients with IC generally urinate many times per day. In moderate cases of IC, patients may void fourteen to eighteen times per day, roughly twice as often as the average person. In severe cases, patients may void twenty-five or more times per day. During a severe flare, it is not uncommon to void every ten to twenty minutes. This is difficult to understand for someone who has not experienced it. The urge is *so* strong, and the pain *so* intense, that IC patients *must* try to void in order to achieve some temporary relief.

One of the hallmarks of IC is getting up to void at night. Although this seems to happen to many women after childbirth and with aging, people with active IC void at least four times a night, and frequently even more often. This interrupts sleep and makes it harder for the body to perform its normal nighttime healing processes. Patterns of urination in IC are abnormal as well. Many times very small amounts of urine are voided, and some patients experience difficulty urinating completely or have painful urination.

A woman with IC may have significant pelvic inflammation and may experience a worsening of symptoms at certain times during her menstrual cycle, indicating that hormones may play a role. Roughly 60–70 percent of women with IC report having pain with intercourse, and in a study examining women with IC/PBS, there appears to be a strong correlation with vulvodynia (for more on this see Chapter 8, "Help with Hormones and Alleviating Feminine Discomfort").[22]

In some patients, complaints of pain with voiding are confined mainly to the urethra. As with more typical cases of IC, there is no evidence of infection and symptoms do not usually resolve with antibiotics or with anti-inflammatory drugs. This type of condition may be diagnosed as "urethral syndrome," and it is usually considered to be a variant of IC (painful bladder syndrome). There are a few other conditions that can cause these symptoms, so it is a good idea to have a thorough workup by a urologist.

It is also extremely common for IC patients to be unable to tolerate eating certain foods, because these foods make symptoms worse and, in some cases, may even cause bladder symptoms. You will learn much more about this very important link between food sensitivities and bladder symptoms in the chapters ahead.

✳ Diagnosis

The American Urological Association (AUA) educates medical providers in the diagnosis and treatment of urological diseases in order to provide the best care for patients. Beginning in 2008, more than a dozen researchers and clinicians met to systematically review decades of IC research studies. Led by The University of Pennsylvania's Dr. Phillip Hanno, the group worked to explore new IC theories and to propose current guidelines for diagnosis. Following peer review, the group's recommendations were approved by the AUA board in January, 2011. Full guidelines can be downloaded from AUANET.org.

The new AUA guidelines define IC as, "An unpleasant sensation (pain, pressure, discomfort) perceived to be related to the urinary bladder, associated with lower urinary tract symptoms of more than six weeks duration, in the absence of infection or other identifiable causes." (This definition was first proposed by the Society for Urodynamics and Female Urology.) The AUA also took into account recent studies exploring related conditions occurring frequently in IC patients and the possibility that IC is part of a family of hypersensitivity disorders with overlapping symptoms, something that many IC patients, as well as clinicians, have long believed to be true. The guidelines also state that, with regard to diagnosis, a review of IC literature yielded "insufficient evidence," and recommendations are therefore based on clinical principles and expert opinion.

The new AUA guidelines urge clinicians to record a complete patient history, to make a very thorough patient examination, and to carefully review results from urinalysis and urine culture. Cytology, a test to look microscopically for abnormal cells in the urine sample, should be done in patients who have microhematuria (an abnormal number of blood cells in the urine) or a history of smoking. The focus

of the basic assessment should be to rule in symptoms that charac-
terize IC, including pain related to bladder filling, urethral pain, and
pain in other areas of the pelvis, including tenderness and trigger
points in the pelvic floor. The basic assessment should also be used to
rule out conditions such as bladder infections, bladder stones, vaginitis, prostatitis, and, in patients with risk factors, bladder cancer. In the
initial patient assessment, it is important for clinicians to record the
patient's baseline voiding pattern; the location, character and severity
of pain; and symptom duration. (A patient voiding diary is helpful,
and the Pain/Urgency/Frequency patient questionnaire, PUF, is also
a useful tool for diagnosis.) The new guidelines also suggest a brief
exam to rule out neurological causes for symptoms such as incomplete bladder emptying and urinary retention, as well as a complete
abdominal and pelvic exam for both male and female patients.

The urine of IC patients often contains a small number of red
blood cells, but reddish-colored urine indicates some amount of active bleeding from injured epithelium or from other areas of the urinary tract, such as the prostate. Although white blood cells may also
be present, the quantity of them isn't usually high enough to indicate
active infection. [This discussion, which has been revised since the
first printing of this book, is continued on page 277.]

※ *Treatment*

Since IC has no single known cause, medical treatment focuses on
helping people to alleviate discomfort and encouraging patients to
live life as normally as possible. Both medical practitioners and patients have struggled with the frustration of treating this disorder,
but the new AUA guidelines should help streamline treatment and
give clinicians effective options for referring patients to chronic pain
specialists when appropriate. Chapter 3 discusses "Traditional Treatments" used in IC.

Throughout this book you will learn many tools and techniques
to use when your bladder pain is flaring. But more importantly, you
will learn how to make significant dietary and lifestyle changes that
can lead to a remission of IC symptoms. Below are some simple yet
effective suggestions. These are discussed in greater detail in Part II,
the recovery portion of this book, and especially in Chapter 4.

- Keep a diet journal, a simple notebook small enough to fit into your purse or jacket pocket, to help you track what foods may be triggering your bladder symptoms. Many IC patients have found that bladder pain can be triggered by eating gluten, as well as by other food allergies and sensitivities. Gluten sensitivity is strongly linked to bladder pain, frequency, and urgency, as well as to chronic inflammation of the bladder and prostate. Bladder pain can also be triggered by eating "extreme foods" — those that are very acidic, very salty, very sweet, or very spicy. In general, all forms of caffeine, including espresso, regular brewed coffee, chocolate, many brands of soft drinks, black tea, and, for some, even green tea, are very irritating to the bladder.

- If you have eaten extreme foods, drinking a few glasses of water can help to flush out your bladder and can dilute the offending substances in your system. You can also try drinking an eight-ounce glass of water with a quarter teaspoon of baking soda stirred into it, especially if you have eaten acidic foods. If you have high blood pressure, first check with your physician about this, as higher amounts of baking soda can result in an increased level of sodium in the blood, potentially raising the blood pressure. Too much baking soda in your glass of water may also taste unpalatable.

- If you seem to have food sensitivities or allergies, try an over-the-counter antihistamine, like Claritin, or a natural antihistamine, like nettle leaf tea. You can carry it with you or keep it in a desk drawer at your office. Antihistamines can help to minimize bladder pain caused by an allergic reaction.

- Bladder pain in some women is triggered by hormonal fluctuations and can often be much more severe at certain times of the month. Your gynecologist may be able to help you if your bladder symptoms worsen with your monthly cycle.

- Pelvic pain and inflammation can often be alleviated by alternating cold packs and heating pads over the pelvic area, or by placing a medicated over-the-counter treatment, such as a Tiger-Balm Patch, over your bladder.

- Chamomile tea is a very useful herbal remedy to help prevent and calm bladder spasms. It is mild and gentle, and it is safe enough for children. You will learn much more about helpful herbal teas throughout the book, and in Appendix B, which covers herbal remedies in detail.

- Omega-3 oils from sources such as flaxseed, fish, borage, black currant, and evening primrose can help alleviate inflammation and pain. Mix one or two tablespoons of flaxseed oil with a little juice, and take before bedtime. Flaxseed oil and most of the other suggested omega-3 oils also come in gel-capsule form.

- To the extent possible, try to determine if anything is acting as an immediate trigger for your IC pain. Drinking coffee, wearing tight jeans, and spending too much time sitting on hard surfaces are some examples. It may be just as important to *stop* doing something that is aggravating your pain as it is to *begin* a new treatment regimen.

FAQs | Interstitial Cystitis

Q: *Is my bladder ever going to get better?*
A: The answer to this question, of course, depends on the cause of your bladder problems. Urologists may tell you that IC can be a progressive disease, although many people do experience remissions lasting from months to years. There are many anecdotal reports of people who have recovered from IC, though, and you may be one of these. Persistence and a positive attitude can make a big difference in your progress.

IC is not alone in causing chronic bladder problems. If you are an older person or a woman who experienced childbirth trauma to the pelvic floor, you may have been told that your stress incontinence is inevitable. But, proper diet, exercise, topical hormone treatments, and physical therapy aimed at pelvic floor rehabilitation can make a difference for you, too. For other disorders that may cause bladder symptoms, refer to Chapter 11, "Medical Conditions and Other Sources of Pelvic Pain or Bladder Symptoms."

Q: *What is double voiding?*
A: Double voiding is the medical term for a pattern in which the

bladder does not empty completely on the first try and you feel a strong urge to void again in about twenty or thirty minutes. This sometimes occurs in people with IC. It can be caused by spasms of the bladder, urethra, or pelvic floor muscles. Your physical therapist or physician may be able to teach you some helpful techniques to deal with this, particularly if you are able to describe your symptoms accurately. Relaxation techniques are often very effective. Antispasmodic medications or herbal preparations may be useful as well. Double voiding is one of the abnormal voiding patterns that sometimes occur in people with IC, and it is an endless source of frustration for the already sleep-deprived.

Q: *Is my bladder capacity shrinking because of my IC?*
A: Over time, IC damages the bladder lining, creating scar tissue. As the scar tissue builds up over many years, it reduces the bladder's natural elasticity, significantly decreasing bladder capacity. One of the goals of any IC treatment plan should be to minimize the damage that creates scar tissue and to help preserve bladder capacity, and therefore quality of life.

Q: *Is my bladder disease inherited?*
A: The jury is still out on this question because we have not yet discovered the precise cause of IC, although there seems to be some agreement on contributing elements. Recently, more researchers are beginning to explore the possibility that heredity may play a part in some forms of IC. Cases have been reported of identical twins with IC, and of mothers and daughters with IC.[24] Recent studies in Denmark indicate a possible genetic tendency for the mental illness schizophrenia, certain autoimmune diseases, and IC to cluster.[25] Another study, at Columbia University, examined disease clusters that include IC, panic disorder, depression, thyroid disorders, and celiac disease. Researchers concluded: "[T]he hypothesis that there is a familial syndrome that may include IC . . . and other disorders of possible autonomic or neuromuscular control deserves further investigation."[26]

❋ *IC and Autoimmune Disorders*

Autoimmune disorders include such well-known diseases as rheumatoid arthritis, type-I diabetes, lupus, and multiple sclerosis. Autoimmune disorders involve a process in which the immune system overreacts, producing cytokines and other inflammatory substances in response to a perceived invasion that mistakenly targets the body's own tissues. In rheumatoid arthritis, the tissue attacked is mainly the joints and connective tissue; in diabetes, it is the pancreas; in multiple sclerosis, it is the nervous system.

Autoimmune disorders and the autoimmune response are major sources of inflammation in the body, and there appear to be clear associations between IC and immune-mediated disorders such as chronic fatigue/fibromyalgia, irritable bowel syndrome, and, most especially, Sjögren's syndrome.[27]

Sjögren's syndrome is a chronic autoimmune disorder in which the immune system attacks the body's moisture-producing glands, including those in the eyes, mouth, respiratory tract, and vagina. Therefore, common symptoms are dry eyes, dry mouth, dry throat, and dry vaginal tissues (among others). The link between Sjögren's syndrome and IC was investigated at a meeting of the International Painful Bladder Foundation in 2006, and a general consensus was reached that both OAB and PBS/IC are known to be associated with Sjögren's syndrome.[28] However, this association was noted much earlier. A small study in 1993 reported finding Sjögren's syndrome in eight out of ten patients with confirmed IC and concluded that IC was a "new" disease occurring in association with Sjögren's syndrome.[29] This is yet another example that supports the theory that IC *is* an autoimmune condition. Certainly, patients with either IC or Sjögren's syndrome should consider being screened for other associated autoimmune disorders, particularly if characteristic symptoms are present.

Similarly, a Finnish study showed that patients with lupus (systemic lupus erythematosus, SLE), another autoimmune disorder, experience significantly more complaints of irritative voiding than matched controls, with the most common complaints being urinary frequency, pain and tenderness just above the pubic bone, and urinary stress incontinence.[30] What is really interesting is the clear association between both Sjögren's syndrome and SLE and another autoimmune disorder, celiac disease. Among those with celiac disease, there is a tenfold increase in risk for developing other autoimmune disorders, including lupus (SLE), Sjögren's syndrome, and rheumatoid arthritis.[31]

Celiac disease, described in Chapter 5, seems to show a strong tendency to affect those with IC. Research studies are being conducted at Baylor College of Medicine and Texas Medical Center examining the link between IC and gluten, which triggers illness in those with celiac disease (see Chapter 5). Some physicians and many patients also consider IC to be an autoimmune disorder, but the scientific evidence isn't yet completely clear. I believe that an autoimmune response is an important and overlooked possible "pathway" to developing IC, and the studies described in the following paragraphs are some of the reasons I believe this to be so.

For more than a decade, we have known that IC and fibromyalgia have a significant overlap in symptoms. Studies in Japan and elsewhere have revealed that at least 11 percent of patients with IC also have fibromyalgia.[32] Studies done at Georgetown University showed that fibromyalgia and IC patients share a pattern of diffuse tenderness in their extremities, increased pain sensitivity compared to healthy control subjects, and symptoms that occur with similar frequency.[33] Although immune system mechanisms have been suspected in fibromyalgia, IC has most often been classified as a "bladder disorder." These studies suggest that there may be a central immune mechanism contributing to both of these disorders.

A 2003 Swedish study examined the possible link between IC and autoimmune disorders in 220 IC patients and determined that an allergy-driven autoimmune response could be involved. Study results showed that allergy was the most common IC-associated condition, with 41 percent of patients with "classic" IC and 47 percent of patients with the nonulcerative form of IC exhibiting hypersensitivity/allergy reactions. The study also found that other autoimmune disorders such as Crohn's and ulcerative colitis were present in "classic" IC patients at *thirty-three times* the prevalence found in the general population![34]

Autoantibodies, or antibodies that react against one's own body, have been found in patients with IC, specifically autoantibodies that react against bladder epithelium. However, it isn't yet clear what role, if any, they play in the disease process. There is a good deal of clinical evidence of possible autoimmune involvement, including the fact that IC tends to affect many more women than men, a fact also true of autoimmune diseases. There are also supporting clinical correlations between IC and other known autoimmune diseases, such as Sjögren's syndrome. Studies done in the Netherlands identified autoantibodies to the muscarinic M3 receptor in patients with Sjögren's. Muscarinic M3 receptors are involved in smooth-muscle contraction. What's really interesting is that cells in the detrusor muscle, which is largely responsible for bladder contraction, contain these M3 receptors. The studies' authors concluded that these autoantibodies to M3 may play an important role in both noninflammatory and inflammatory aspects of IC.[35]

Interestingly, Sjögren's is one of the more common autoimmune disorders linked to celiac disease, in which the gluten protein triggers an autoimmune response in the body against a variety of the body's tissues. The connection between gluten intolerance and IC, including a possible mechanism of injury to the bladder wall, will be discussed in greater detail in the chapters that lie ahead.

In the past, few effective treatments existed for autoimmune disorders. Newer treatments include TNF (tissue necrosis factor) blockers, which help prevent damage to the body's tissues and suppress the immune system. Some people have had success with complementary-medicine treatments for autoimmune disorders; these can be explored with a naturopath or a practitioner of traditional Chinese medicine (TCM). A gluten-free diet may also be beneficial in treating many other autoimmune disorders, including MS, rheumatoid arthritis, and, of course, celiac disease.

❊ Growing Awareness

Thanks to the efforts of health professionals like the Interstitial Cystitis Association's Dr. Vicki Ratner; Interstitial Cystitis Network founder Jill Osborne; the IC Puzzle's Amrit Willis, RN; author and educator Gaye Sandler; and others who have dedicated themselves to education and greater awareness of IC, this frustrating disorder is finally beginning to receive more attention from the scientific community. Research is currently being conducted by six research centers throughout the country in a program funded by the NIH (National Institutes of Health; see Resources). Hopefully it will bear fruit in the form of viable new treatments for IC and OAB.

Urinary Tract Problems in Men

Men can develop both IC and overactive bladder, although both seem to be far more common in women. Men can be diagnosed with CPP, also usually referred to in men as CPPS. The wonderful resource book *A Headache in the Pelvis: A New Understanding and Treatment for Prostatitis and Chronic Pelvic Pain Syndromes*, by Drs. Wise and Anderson, addresses these problems in men. Beyond some musculoskeletal disorders, chronic pelvic pain in men is often caused by or associated with inflammation of the prostate gland, called prostatitis.

Prostatitis

The prostate gland's job is to secrete seminal fluid, the milky substance that, combined with sperm, makes up semen. As mentioned earlier, the prostate's location, surrounding the urethra, is often problematic later in life, as most men undergo at least some degree of prostate enlargement, which can constrict the flow of urine through the urethra.

Inflammation of the prostate gland may result from a urinary tract infection or from urethritis (inflammation of the urethra), or it may be present in the absence of identified infection and may be diagnosed as asymptomatic inflammation. Although many people do not know much about prostatitis, about half of all men will be affected by it at some point in their lives. This painful and frustrating health problem is responsible for two million visits to doctors annually in the United States.

Prostatitis affects men of all ages, from men in their early twenties to seniors. Those with a history of sexually transmitted infections (STIs) are at increased risk for prostatitis, as are men with a history of UTI and men over age fifty.

❊ Symptoms

The most commonly reported symptom of prostatitis, occurring in roughly two-thirds of patients, is pain, located in the perineum (the area between the scrotum and anus), in the rectum, or just above the pubic bone. Pain can be referred to the penis as well. Other possible symptoms include severe urinary frequency, incomplete voiding (related to partial obstruction of the urethra), and erectile dysfunction.

In severe cases of prostatitis, when inflammation leads to obstruction of urine flow, kidney infection can result, causing great discomfort and eventually becoming life-threatening sepsis. If you are suffering symptoms of prostatitis and begin experiencing nausea and vomiting, cramping, pain in your mid-back or side, a fever, or chills, seek immediate medical help.

❊ *Diagnosis*

Diagnosis is based on a combination of reported symptoms and physical examination. Two initial urine specimens are taken. Then the doctor manually palpates the prostate gland through the barrier of the rectal wall in a procedure known as a digital rectal exam. This is the much-joked-about, dreaded "rubber-glove" exam. Very simply, the examiner inserts a lubricated, gloved finger into the rectum and feels the shape and size of the prostate gland. The exam will also show whether the prostate is tender or inflamed. During this process, the prostate gland can be massaged to release prostatic secretions, which are then placed in a third specimen container and examined for the presence of white blood cells, PIAs (prostatic inflammatory aggregates — a sign of acute inflammation), and bacteria. The results are compared to those from the previous two samples to help locate the source of the infection, if any. Doctors are sometimes cautious about this procedure, because in the case of acute bacterial prostatitis it can spread the bacteria. (Semen may also be examined, especially when bacterial infection is suspected.)

A 2005 Scandinavian study found that, in addition to the bacteria commonly associated with urinary tract infection, various species of mycoplasma organisms were seen significantly more frequently in the semen of patients with prostatitis than in the control group.[36] Recently, research has begun to focus on the possible role of another organism, *Chlamydia pneumoniae*, in chronic prostatitis. (See Chapter 10, "The Embattled Body: Dealing with Infectious Microorganisms.")

When neither infection nor another organ-specific cause can be found, and symptoms persist, a diagnosis of prostatodynia may be made. The term prostatodynia (also known as prostadynia) is now used synonymously with CPPS.

☀ *Treatment*

The goals of treatment in prostatitis are to reduce discomfort and decrease inflammation. In the case of acute bacterial prostatitis, antibiotics are the treatment of choice. Pain medications, anti-inflammatories, and drugs such as Flomax (tamsulosin hydrochloride) may also be prescribed. Several recent studies have indicated that at least a third of men with prostatitis have their symptoms resolve within one year.

"Complementary" treatments for prostatitis include using the nutritional supplement bromelain for its anti-inflammatory properties; using the herbs saw palmetto, nettle root, and pygeum to decrease inflammation and improve urine flow (see Appendix B, on herbal remedies); and taking 30 mg of zinc daily. Zinc is important to prostate health and also helps reduce the risk of infections. Zinc taken on an empty stomach may cause slight nausea, so take it with a meal.

| Sidebar | **Urine Retention** |

Urine retention can be a result of incomplete bladder emptying or a result of constriction. In normal urination, the bladder empties completely, but when there is a problem with the nerves that control the bladder, as in spinal cord injury, multiple sclerosis, and other neurological disorders, some amount of urine remains in the bladder, increasing the risk of developing infection. Obstruction of the urinary tract is also a cause of urine retention. Obstruction can be partial or complete, and chronic or acute. Major causes of partial obstruction are prostatitis, whether associated with UTI or not; benign prostatic hypertrophy (BPH), an enlargement of the prostate; and bladder neck stenosis, or narrowing of the bladder neck. But another, often-overlooked cause is certain medications that can cause urine retention or even a sudden inability to urinate. It is important to pay attention to the warnings on both prescription and over-the-counter medications. They usually read something like, "If you suffer from an enlarged prostate or BPH, this medication may cause an inability to void."

(cont'd.)

Unfortunately, the list of medications that can cause urine retention is lengthy, and includes common medications such as antihistamines, decongestants, tricyclic antidepressants, and medications for the treatment of Parkinson's disease. Another class of problematic medications is narcotic analgesics, including morphine. Benzodiazepines, which include the antianxiety medications Valium and Xanax, and the sleep aid Restoril, also have the potential to cause urine retention. If you suffer from BPH, ask your pharmacist for a complete list of medications that can cause urine retention or have your pharmacist screen any prescribed medications for this potential side effect.

Chronic Prostatitis (CP, or CPPS)

For some patients, inflammation of the prostate becomes chronic and can result in a condition known as CP, sometimes referred to as CPPS. In the past, this condition has also been known as chronic nonbacterial prostatitis and, less commonly, as prostatodynia. As many as 10 percent of adult men may have genetic factors that predispose them to developing this disorder, but larger studies are needed to confirm this figure.[37] Other factors that may play a part in the development of this disorder include neurogenic inflammation, stress-driven adrenal dysfunction, and myofascial pain syndrome. Throughout this book you will learn in detail about these contributors to chronic pain and inflammation, and you will learn the tools and techniques you need to gain control over chronic pelvic pain.

❊ Symptoms

According to the excellent book *A Headache in the Pelvis*, common symptoms of chronic (nonbacterial) prostatitis include intermittent or chronic pain, intermittent or chronic urinary symptoms (including reduced flow, frequency, urgency, and pain with urination), possible sexual dysfunction, and anxiety, depression, or both.[38]

Postejaculatory pain is very common, affecting nearly three-quarters of men with chronic prostatitis/chronic pelvic pain syndrome, and it is specific enough to help distinguish between CPPS and other chronic conditions such as BPH.[39] (In contrast, some men experience pain *relief* following ejaculation.) In addition to the obvious discomfort and dysfunction related to prostatitis, chronic inflammation can lead to scarring and eventually to an increased risk for developing both BPH and prostate cancer.

❊ Diagnosis

A diagnosis of CP or CPPS can be made when there is no evidence of infection, and the symptoms described above have been present for a period of three months or more. Symptoms don't need to be constant to meet diagnostic criteria but rather may come and go. Prior to 2003, chronic bacterial infection was still regarded as a major cause of CPPS, but a University of Washington study found that about one-third of both CP patients and men without prostate complaints had equal numbers of similar bacteria colonizing their prostates, suggesting a lesser role for infection.[40]

❊ Treatment

Treatment with antibiotics is ineffective in nonbacterial, chronic prostatitis.[41] This condition requires a different approach: If you've been diagnosed with CPPS, examine your lifestyle, including diet, work habits, and exercise routines, as a possible source of chronic inflammation. Perhaps a pattern will emerge. Maybe you developed your first symptoms after that hundred-mile bike ride, or when you switched from site foreman, an on-your-feet job, to project manager, a desk job. Think about your overall health. Everything is connected — one's appearance, skin integrity, weight, mood, and energy level reflect what is going on inside one's body.

A newer treatment strategy, known as the Stanford Protocol, involves relaxation, behavioral therapy, and myofascial trigger point release (see Chapter 7). This approach to treating CPPS was developed by, among others, Rodney Anderson, MD; David Wise, PhD; and physical therapist Tim Sawyer. There is some evidence that anxiety plays a role in the development, and certainly the management, of CPPS. The results of the Stanford group's study showed that *more than half* of the patients who participated in this treatment program improved. These clinicians now have a successful track record and believe that their protocol can relieve CPPS and urinary symptoms as well as or better than traditional methods. For more information on this topic, go to the website www.pelvicpainhelp.com, or read their book *A Headache in the Pelvis*.

To maintain prostate health, it is also important to follow a healthy diet and to maintain a healthy weight, as obesity is an important risk factor. Men with prostate symptoms should also be encouraged to drink adequate quantities of water and to eliminate food sensitivities (see below). In particular, there is an association between prostatitis and gluten sensitivity, just as there is between IC and gluten sensitivity. In fact, the two pelvic pain disorders share so many similarities that some researchers feel they are variants of the same disease.[42] As early as 2001, research showed that nearly 70 percent of men with chronic nonbacterial prostatitis and CPPS have evidence of IC when they undergo cystoscopy, suggesting that IC in men is often misdiagnosed as nonbacterial prostatitis, and that chronic pelvic pain in men may be the chief characteristic of IC.[43] In 2007, IC/PBS and CP/CPPS began to be grouped under the umbrella term urologic chronic pelvic pain syndromes (UCPPS).

While researching the many varieties of bladder and pelvic disorders, including chronic prostatitis, when I looked for a link to gluten sensitivity, it wasn't difficult to find. There are many reports that patients with gluten intolerance or celiac disease suffer severe flares in their chronic pelvic pain symptoms after eating gluten.[44] Likewise, there are many anecdotal reports of men who have been able to resolve their chronic prostatitis symptoms by eliminating gluten. Here, Marc M., a naprapathic physician (DN)*, shares his story:

CASE STUDY: *Marc's Story*

I thought you might be interested in my case, which comes from a male perspective. I've suffered from IBS, frequent urination, and chronic prostatitis for about twenty-five years, since I was a teenager. I'm also severely dairy intolerant, following a life-threatening bout of chicken pox at age thirty. I've been to numerous doctors, including gastroenterologists, and have been through the gamut of treatments for noninflammatory bowel disease. However, I personally knew little about nutrition or holistic medicine until I met my wife. I'm from an Italian background, so having wheat/gluten on the table three times

---

* Naprapathy is a method of healing that works through the connective tissues, including ligaments, tendons, and muscles, to release tensions that cause structural imbalance in the body.

a day was typical in my family. My wife had done a lot of nutritional work, and she helped me understand how this type of diet was affecting my body. Going gluten-free has brought me nearly complete (99.9 percent) relief from IBS symptoms, and it has definitely helped resolve my chronic prostatitis as well. I've also done some detoxification with specific products to support my immune system and have done some bioidentical hormone treatment under the guidance of a physician with a functional medicine approach. I had some nocturia previously, but now I can sleep through the night unless I overindulge in fluids during the day—a significant improvement!

What You Can Do Now

The most important thing you can do now is to find the best health practitioner you can—one who meets your specific needs—and then obtain an accurate diagnosis for your condition (or conditions). Remember, it is very common for several pelvic pain conditions to occur together. It is also sometimes valuable to have *several* different practitioners on your "health-care team," for example, an ob-gyn, a naturopathic physician, and a physical therapist. Each of these health-care specialties can complement the others and work together synergistically toward a more rapid recovery. Once you've obtained an accurate diagnosis and have found a practitioner you feel comfortable working with, you can move on to learning the valuable tools for managing your symptoms, found in Chapter 4.

3

Traditional
Treatments

If you have been diagnosed with interstitial cystitis (IC)/painful bladder syndrome (PBS), overactive bladder (OAB), or chronic prostatitis (CP)/chronic pelvic pain syndrome (CPPS), and you are being treated by a urologist practicing mainstream medicine, you will most likely be offered medications in several categories. This chapter reviews each of these medications and their possible side effects, as well as other common allopathic treatments for these conditions.

Medications
for IC/PBS and CPP

Medications for treating chronic bladder problems fall into several broad categories: drugs to repair the bladder lining, drugs to treat the allergy component of IC, pain medications, antispasmodics, and antianxiety medications.

Elmiron: A Synthetic Glycosaminoglycan
for Bladder-Lining Repair

Elmiron (pentosan polysulfate sodium), a drug developed to help repair the bladder lining, is the only currently approved medication used specifically to treat interstitial cystitis. Is it the answer to your problems? Maybe. Many patients don't experience relief from their IC pain for the first three to four months after starting on Elmiron, and a decrease in urinary frequency may take even longer. (Patients are encouraged to stay on their drug therapy for at least three to six months before making the decision to stop treatment.) Some short-term clinical studies have shown treatment with Elmiron to result in improvement in symptoms in roughly one third of patients at the end of six months of therapy. However, in a long-term study, 97 IC patients were followed for approximately nine years (from 1987 through 1995). The results showed that at the end of the study far fewer than a third (6.2 percent to 18.7 percent) of the patients continued to benefit from treatment with Elmiron.[1]

While the success rate isn't as high as we'd ideally like, some patients do enjoy a much better quality of life with the use of Elmiron, but it can come at a price — literally. Elmiron is a very, very expensive drug, and you will need to check with your insurance company to make sure it is fully covered. If you are not insured, you may be unable to afford this drug. One option is to contact the manufacturer; they may offer to provide the drug for you at a reduced cost if you qualify for one of their special Patient Assistance Programs (PAPs).

✳ *Action*

Elmiron is a mucopolysaccharide that helps to repair the protective GAG (glycosaminoglycan) layer lining the bladder mucosa. (Mucopolysaccharides are long-chained molecules composed of sugars, creating a jelly-like substance commonly found in mucous secretions and in the fluid that cushions joints.) The drug initially was thought to hold much promise, and it has been able to help many people. I also appreciate the fact that pharmaceutical companies are actively conducting research on medications to treat IC, evidence of the disorder's significant presence in our population. That being said, I believe that future drug research may yield more effective medications that have fewer significant side effects and are more affordable.

✳ *Side Effects*

For many patients, Elmiron's most common side effects are minor gastrointestinal discomfort and headaches. A small percentage of patients experienced patchy hair loss, but hair grew back when they stopped taking the drug. Elmiron can also have significant side effects, including severe headaches, skin rash, weight gain, and sun sensitivity. It is important to note that 52 percent of the participants dropped out of the Physician's Usage Study before the end of the recommended treatment period.[2] Side effects of concern are increased bruising and, especially, *increased risk of bleeding*. In an eight-month-long study, 6.3 percent of 128 patients reportedly experienced bleeding from the rectum.[3]

Although researchers have not found any negative interactions between Elmiron and other medications, *Elmiron may affect liver function, so your physician will need to monitor your progress*. Elmiron has not been tested in pregnant women; therefore, it isn't recommended for use during pregnancy.

Atarax (Hydroxyzine): A Powerful Antihistamine

Atarax (hydroxyzine hydrochloride) is a strong antihistamine that also has both pain-relieving and sedating properties. It can reduce the effect of irritating histamines in the urine, help reduce pain, and improve sleep. It is dangerous to take hydroxyzine before driving or operating machinery, which makes it impractical to take on a regular basis when you do need to drive, work, and be mentally alert. The sedating effect is less noticeable after you have taken hydroxyzine for a while, but is unlikely to go away completely.

Some physicians recommend over-the-counter antihistamines such as Claritin, Zyrtec, Tagamet, or even Benadryl in place of hydroxyzine. An even better substitute may be nettle leaf tea or capsules. However, tracking down your own food allergies is the best option of all.

❊ Action

Hydroxyzine is thought to work by blocking histamine, a substance produced by the body during an allergic response. Its calming and analgesic effect may work by inhibiting other natural substances such as acetylcholine and serotonin, or by acting directly on certain parts of the brain.

☀ *Side Effects*

Frequent side effects include drowsiness, dizziness, blurred vision, dry mouth, and headache. Rare and more serious side effects that have been reported include anxiety, confusion, hallucinations, shaking tremors, decreased and or painful urination, difficulty urinating (urinary hesitancy), and vision changes. *Very serious reactions can include irregular heartbeat, seizures, and difficulty breathing caused by anaphylaxis, a life-threatening reaction.*

Multiple sources cite hydroxyzine as "not recommended" for use during pregnancy, especially in the first trimester. Likewise, it is not recommended to use hydroxyzine while breast-feeding.

Elavil (Amitriptyline): An Antidepressant Used to Treat Chronic Pain

While antidepressants may have a bad rap among people with chronic pain, it is important to know that a physician does not usually suggest an antidepressant as a Band-Aid to make you feel better, or because he or she thinks your disease is "all in your head." Antidepressants can have a *very real* effect on enabling the body to handle pain more effectively and are often prescribed to treat chronic pain. One of them is Elavil (amitriptyline hydrochloride), an oldie but goodie. It is very inexpensive and has manageable side effects for many people, although higher doses may be associated with weight gain.

Elavil, a tricyclic antidepressant, is used to treat depression and other mood disorders in dosages up to 75 mg. But it is also used, in doses as low as 10 to 25 mg, to effectively treat chronic nerve pain, including disorders such as interstitial cystitis and migraine, often in conjunction with other medications (see below). Those who have been unable to tolerate the sedating side effects of amitriptyline may have been placed on too high a dose. A clinical trial begun in 2003 is studying the effectiveness of amitriptyline in treating IC/PBS.[4] The results of the study were unavailable at the time of publication.

☀ *Action*

Amitriptyline is believed to block nerve signals that trigger pain in the bladder. It may also decrease muscle spasms in the bladder, helping to reduce frequent urination.

❊ Side Effects

Amitriptyline may cause drowsiness, dizziness, increased sun sensitivity, blurred vision, orthostatic hypotension (dizziness upon rising from a sitting or lying position), dry mouth, and restlessness. Rare and more serious side effects can include irregular heartbeat, difficulty urinating (urinary hesitancy), nightmares, ringing in the ears, uncoordinated movements, fainting, and excessive drowsiness. *Very serious side effects also include rash, itching, swelling, and trouble breathing.*

Amitriptyline interacts with many other prescription medications; some over-the-counter medications, including cough and cold remedies; and the herb St. John's wort.

It is important to know that amitriptyline should be started at the lowest dose possible and gradually increased to the lowest effective dose. It may take two to three weeks before the full benefit of this medication becomes apparent, and the medication should never be withdrawn or stopped suddenly. Tapering down is necessary to prevent severe side effects. Note that the onset for the muscle-relaxing and pain-relieving effects of this medication may differ from the typical onset for its effectiveness as an antidepressant, as a different action is involved.

In studies reviewed by McQuay and others at the University of Oxford, it was reported that "[T]ricyclics seem to be the only (antidepressant) drugs of proven benefit [for chronic neuropathic (nerve) pain]."[5]

A newer antidepressant, Cymbalta, is thought to be a good choice for chronic pain management in fibromyalgia and nerve pain, and was recently approved by the FDA for this purpose. The antidepressant Paxil (paroxitine), a selective serotonin reuptake inhibitor (SSRI), may be worth discussing with your physician for short-term use, as it has a relatively long track record, favorable results in the Oxford study cited above, and a low rate of urinary side effects. But there are also alternatives to antidepressants, including exercise, relaxation and other lifestyle changes, and herbal remedies.

This combination of three drugs — Elmiron, an antihistamine, and an antidepressant — is a common pharmaceutical approach to treating IC.

Neurontin (Gabapentin): A Medication for Chronic Nerve Pain

This medication is classified as an anticonvulsant—a drug used to prevent seizures—but is also sometimes prescribed as a mood stabilizer in the treatment of bipolar disorder. It has pain-blocking properties, and it is used to treat shingles (herpes zoster) and foot pain caused by diabetic neuropathy. Some chronic pain specialists and neurologists have prescribed it in the treatment of both severe IC and fibromyalgia, although these are considered "off-label" uses.[6]

❊ Action

Neurontin works on neuropathic pain, which involves the misfiring of nerves. Symptoms of neuropathic pain often go beyond normal pain sensations and can include burning, tingling, numbness, weakness, and sensitivity to light touch. According to Daniel Carr, MD, medical director of Tufts New England Center, "Although chronic pain isn't always neuropathic, a lot of chronic pain conditions are now recognized as having a neuropathic component."[7] Neurontin is thought to help alleviate this type of pain by slowing the conduction of nerve impulses from the spinal cord to more distant body parts.

Another possible mechanism for Neurontin's effect on neuropathic pain is that it may decrease the activity of a neurotransmitter called substance P. Substance P does two things: It carries pain messages through the nervous system, and it stimulates inflammation, both of which can affect chronic pain. Many patients with IC and/or fibromyalgia have elevated levels of substance P.

The individual response to Neurontin in the treatment of chronic pain appears to be highly variable, with some patients experiencing an immediate improvement in pain levels with few side effects, some who need to work up to a much higher dose for effective results, and others who receive little benefit.

Neurontin isn't considered to be habit-forming, and doctors believe that it works best when taken at regular intervals so that a steady blood level is maintained. That said, I have found it effective to take Neurontin occasionally for relief of occipital nerve pain from a pinched nerve at the back of my neck—I just don't drive after I've taken it, as I have noted it does affect me cognitively.

❋ Side Effects

Common side effects include blurred vision; dizziness; drowsiness; swelling of hands, feet, or lower legs; trembling; and unusual tiredness or weakness. Less-common side effects include diarrhea, frequent urination, headache, lowered blood pressure, nausea, noise in the ears, difficulty thinking and sleeping, vomiting, and weight gain. *The following symptoms always require notification of your doctor: unsteady gait, uncontrolled eye-rolling, depression, irritability, memory loss, fever, chills, lower-back or side pain, and painful or difficult urination.*

Neurontin isn't for use during pregnancy. Due to reduced kidney function in the elderly, Neurontin should be used at the lowest dose possible, and due to the possibility of significant side effects, it should be used only if it is the sole (or best) treatment option available for a given patient.

For patients with IC there may be another disadvantage to using Neurontin: In some people, it seems to *cause* bladder pain. This problem was brought to light by a registered nurse named Marilyn Kerr, who has both IC and fibromyalgia. Although Ms. Kerr initially experienced a relief of aches and pains (her fibromyalgia symptoms) and a sense of well-being after beginning treatment with Neurontin, in a very short time she experienced increased bladder pain.[8] She worked with Pfizer, the drug's manufacturer, to locate other IC patients with a similar experience; I don't know the results of her search.

❋ Interactions

Neurontin's possible interactions with other drugs are best discussed with your pharmacist. It is known to interact with other anticonvulsants, naproxen (a nonsteroidal anti-inflammatory drug [NSAID] used as a pain reliever), Vicodin, and morphine.

Lyrica (Pregalbin): Another Medication for Treating Chronic Pain

Lyrica, a newer drug, is used in ways similar to Neurontin, but despite the good press it initially received not all patients tolerate it well. Lyrica is used to treat neuropathic pain associated with diabetic neuropathy and postherpetic neuralgia from shingles. Like Neurontin, it is used to treat partial onset seizures. It is one of the few drugs approved by the FDA to treat the pain of fibromyalgia, and some pain specialists have had good results treating IC with it as well. It can be taken with or without food. Unlike Neurontin, there is some risk of addiction, and physicians should carefully evaluate patients with a history of drug abuse before prescribing Lyrica. It is a Schedule V controlled substance, meaning it is recognized to have some addictive potential.

❅ *Action*

Lyrica is believed to affect the central nervous system, reducing the level of perceived pain, but the exact mechanism of action is unknown. Studies with animal models suggest that Lyrica reduces hyperexcitability by decreasing the release of the neurotransmitters glutamate, substance P (involved in inflammation), and norepinephrine.

❅ *Side Effects*

In clinical studies, 14 percent of all patients who were treated with Lyrica stopped taking it due to adverse reactions, including dizziness, sleepiness, blurred vision, ataxia (difficulty walking, uncoordinated gait), and other visual disturbances, and abnormal thinking.[9] In the studies, 6 percent of people reported peripheral edema (swelling of hands, feet, and lower legs). In addition, *patients taking Lyrica have an increased risk of developing angioedema — severe swelling of the face, tongue, lips, gums, neck, throat, and larynx. Since angioedema can be life-threatening, anyone with these symptoms should contact medical help immediately and discontinue taking Lyrica.*

Lyrica may cause weight gain. Clinical trial results showed that 9 percent of patients taking this medication experienced an average 7 percent weight gain.[10]

Other serious considerations include increased creatine kinase (an enzyme that, when elevated, indicates tissue damage), decreased platelet counts, and skin lesions. Lyrica isn't recommended for use during pregnancy. Due to reduced renal clearance in the elderly, Lyrica should be used at the lowest dose possible, and it should be used only if it is the sole (or best) treatment option.

Users of Lyrica should never discontinue the drug abruptly but should taper off slowly over a period of at least one week. It is best to discuss discontinuing any medication with your physician and pharmacist.

Narcotics

Doctors may offer to prescribe narcotic pain medications to help you manage your severe pain. It is important to know that opiates are among the *least effective* medications for chronic pain, they are addictive, and they produce other common side effects such as severe constipation. It is also possible to build up a tolerance to opiate narcotics, causing a need to take higher and higher doses for them to be effective. For these reasons, many doctors are reluctant to prescribe narcotic pain medications. Still, your pain should never be ignored. Narcotics can be used with caution to treat flares, and as a temporary bridge until you are able to recover your bladder health, but are not a good choice to use on a regular basis unless there is no other solution. If your physician cannot come up with any alternatives to continued narcotic use, you should consider asking for a referral to a chronic pain specialist, who can probably offer you a broader range of options for control of chronic pain.

Antianxiety Medications, Muscle Relaxants, and Antispasmodics

Again, if your physician prescribes any of these classes of drugs, it is important to be assured that she or he isn't trying to turn you into an addict. Antispasmodics, muscle relaxants, and antianxiety medications are meant to be used "as needed," in order to control severe flare-ups in bladder pain, spasms, and the extreme anxiety that can go along with these symptoms.

These drugs may include baclofen (Lioresal) and alprazolam (Xanax). Baclofen, which is a derivative of gamma-aminobutyric acid (GABA), is used to treat spasticity of the skeletal muscles, which may be useful in cases of pelvic floor dysfunction with muscle spasms. Xanax, a benzodiazepine (related to Valium), is commonly used to treat diagnosed anxiety disorders. In addition to reducing the anxiety that comes with chronic pain, sleeplessness, and flares, Xanax seems to have a relaxant effect on the smooth muscles, and thus may be useful for bladder spasms. Both of these drugs have significant side effects, and they should be used *very carefully*. Seek guidance from your pharmacist and your physician or other practitioner to develop a treatment plan that works for you. In some cases, I believe these drugs can be appropriate for short-term symptom management, especially in IC. Still, alternative options exist that may eliminate the need for these types of medications. For example, there are many herbal remedies that help to treat anxiety and promote relaxation. (Also, see especially Chapter 7, which includes sections on relaxation and exercises for pelvic floor dysfunction, and Chapter 12, which introduces some effective complementary therapeutic techniques.)

Other prescription drugs in this grouping may include Flomax (tamsulosin), to help increase urine flow, and Ditropan (oxybutynin), to help with bladder spasms. "Urinary antispasmodics" are also commonly suggested for patients with OAB and sometimes IC. These include Detrol (tolterodine), Vesicare (solifenacin), Sanctura (trospium), Toviaz (fesoterodine fumarate), and Enablex (darifenacin). Of these, Sanctura appears to be one of the most effective and tolerable. These medications may be useful for treating OAB, but they are less useful for IC, especially over time. Some patients using these medications may experience difficulty urinating or suffer from urinary hesitancy — a particularly annoying, stress-producing symptom that occurs with many anticholinergics and bladder relaxants. The most common side effects are dry mouth and constipation; other side effects may include blurred vision, drowsiness, and decreased sweating. These drugs should not be used when drinking alcohol. In my experience, this class of medications, while helpful for OAB, is not very useful in treating IC, especially if you suffer from urinary hesitancy, or difficulty starting a stream of urine, or if you experience pain with a full bladder, as most people with IC do.

Natural herbal teas such as marshmallow root, slippery elm, plantain, and linden flower may be good substitutes for the drug phenazopyridine hydrochloride (name brand Pyridium, and also contained in some over-the-counter remedies), often prescribed to reduce discomfort and irritation during urination. Herbal teas do not have the harsh side effects of pharmaceuticals, and they may feel soothing to inflamed urethral tissue and comforting to the stomach.

As a registered nurse, I have worked with the medical community in conventional hospital settings for many years. I know that drugs work and that they save many lives. However, I can tell you that I personally have had rather alarming experiences with several conventional IC drugs, including Elmiron, hydroxyzine, and Detrol. As I educated myself about IC and developed my own self-treatment plan, based on diet, lifestyle, and the use of gentle herbal teas, I found good substitutes for all the prescription medications I had formerly used. In the process, I have saved money and avoided the impact that long-term use of those medications would have had on my liver and kidneys, which have the job of processing toxic substances. You may also be able to make this transition.

Over-the-Counter Pain Medications

The over-the-counter pain medications acetaminophen and ibuprofen are not strong enough to handle the severe pain of IC for most people. Ibuprofen and other NSAIDs may even provoke symptoms in people with sensitive, fragile bladder linings.

Invasive Methods of Treatment

Although the following mainstays of conventional IC treatment provide relief for some people, they do little to get IC sufferers on the road to complete recovery because they don't address the condition *holistically*. Treating the symptoms will only get you so far. Some people are fortunate to have a short period of remission following a series of hydrodistentions or bladder instillations. The rule to keep in mind with these treatments is that some people will get better, some will get temporarily worse, and some will experience no change in the level or character of their symptoms.

Bladder Instillation

This treatment, also referred to as intravesical therapy, involves instilling various "cocktails" of medications into the bladder via a catheter. A standard bladder instillation, or "cocktail," combines lidocaine (a local anesthetic), sodium bicarbonate, and either Elmiron or heparin (which are molecularly similar).[11] The treatment needs to be repeated at regular intervals, which are determined by your physician based on your response or progress.

More recently, studies have shown the effectiveness of several new therapies. Chondroitin sulfate is a GAG, the same type of substance that helps to protect the mucosal lining of the bladder. For years, chondroitin sulfate has been instilled in the bladders of IC patients in both Europe and Canada, but not in the United States. Research conducted in the United States, however, has recently shown promise for chondroitin sulfate to aid in the repair of the damaged surface of bladder epithelium in IC patients.[12] Due it its high binding capacity with bladder epithelium, it helps to "plug the holes" and to decrease permeability.

Hyaluronic acid is another GAG present in the mucous layer lining the bladder epithelium. A synthetic version, marketed as the drug Cystistat, has performed fairly well in clinical studies, either alone or in conjunction with chondroitin sulfate.[13] Further studies are needed to determine if long-term treatment is necessary and if it would yield similar results. There have been some indications that the effectiveness of hyaluronic acid in healing the bladder lining may decline slightly over time.

Another study reported at the 2009 meeting of the American Urological Association concerned bladder instillation of liposomes, tiny globules of fat. The study demonstrated that a liposomal instillation known as LP08 was effective in helping to protectively coat the bladder lining, thereby helping to prevent injury. This study was conducted on rat models, but showed that the subjects receiving instillations of liposomes were able to keep their bladder lining intact, while subjects receiving only saline instillations were not.[14]

Other ingredients in bladder-instillation cocktails can include anesthetic solutions, steroids to reduce inflammation, or Rimso (DMSO). DMSO, or dimethyl sulfoxide, is an older approach that some physicians continue to use. But many patients who initially showed positive responses to DMSO later relapsed, and the treatment has also been linked to damage to the bladder muscle, including triggering intense, persistent muscle contractions, even at the

FDA-approved dosage.[15] There are certainly less invasive options to consider. For example, taking the inexpensive over-the-counter supplement MSM (methylsulfonylmethane), an organic form of sulfur known to help with inflammation, may yield a similar effect, without the possibility of damage to the bladder muscle.

Bladder instillations are often done in the physician's office, but it may be possible to learn to do them yourself at home. This is an especially convenient option for those undergoing long-term treatment.

Bladder Hydrodistention

This procedure is exactly what it sounds like. The bladder is distended, or inflated, with liquid, usually a saline solution combined with specific medications. It is used as both a diagnostic test and initial therapy. This is because up to 25 percent of people with IC/PBS have noted at least a temporary improvement in symptoms after a bladder hydrodistention was performed to help diagnose their condition. Temporary bladder distention may increase capacity and interfere with pain signals transmitted by nerves in the bladder.[16]

Although symptoms may initially worsen for four to forty-eight hours after distention, they should return to baseline levels or begin to improve within two to four weeks. The effect lasts for variable amounts of time in different people, but as a general rule may last for up to three to six months.[17]

The AUA guidelines released in 2011 now caution practitioners about offering hydrodistentions routinely, and recommend they be considered only if first- and second- line treatments, including patient education, self-care, stress management, physical therapy, pain management, and oral medications, have not provided relief. The guidelines further recommend only low pressure, short-duration hydrodistention, in order to reduce the risk of bladder rupture. The AUA 2011 guidelines cite several valid reasons for cystoscopy with hydrodistention: First, the cystoscopy can help to identify other potential causes for bladder symptoms; second, hydrodistention allows the examiner to stage disease and confirm reduced capacity resulting from fibrosis (scarring); and third, cytoscopy may identify Hunner's lesions or ulcers. If such abnormalities are found, they can then be treated appropriately *before* the bladder is distended. Hunner's ulcers can be more easily identified when distention leads to increased mucosal cracking and bleeding.

Physical Therapy

Your physician may offer you physical therapy, or you may have to request it, but either way, getting a prescription for six to twelve weeks of specialized physical therapy is a very good idea that can pay big dividends. If you are not yet seeing a physical therapist (PT), consider asking your physician to recommend one who specializes in either women's health or pelvic floor rehabilitation (see also the section in Chapter 7 on pelvic floor dysfunction).

At your first visit, you may have to undergo a physical exam that can feel invasive, as the PT checks for proper internal alignment; she or he will also check the function of the delicate muscles surrounding the vagina, rectum, groin, and pelvic floor. Once your PT diagnoses any specific problems and develops a treatment plan to help you regain normal function, you'll begin regular sessions of physical therapy. You'll usually also be given a set of exercises to do at home between visits. Using a biofeedback technique, your PT can teach you to recognize and release the tension in your pelvic floor muscles and can address any other issues that might be related to your urological dysfunction, including, possibly, birth trauma, sexual trauma, or even childhood abuse (see PTSD and pelvic pain in Chapter 7).

For a look into what physical therapy may offer you, check out the websites listed in Resources under "Pelvic Floor Dysfunction."

Although this approach may not work for everyone, I know of many women who consider themselves healed after committing to a course of physical therapy aimed at pelvic floor rehabilitation. There will be a more in-depth discussion of pelvic floor therapy in Chapter 7.

Treatment by a Chronic Pain Specialist

Assessing, diagnosing, and treating CPP, including IC, can be complicated. But because the disorder is fairly common, some chronic pain practitioners specialize in such treatment. CPP specialists often practice a multidisciplinary approach involving a team of care providers, including nurse practitioners, physical therapists, massage therapists, urologists, gynecologists, and neurologists. This team approach has a research basis behind it: As discussed earlier, CPP frequently has more than one cause, and usually a combination of three or more causes, all of which are better addressed with a multidisciplinary approach. With regard to IC, I would certainly like to see a nutritionist or nurse educator included, because diet has a great impact on this disorder for many people.

A chronic pain specialist may offer you longer-term pain relief in the form of nerve blocks (an injection that interferes with pain signals to the brain, while providing some local anesthetic to the area affected) or even implanted pain-medication pumps.[18] This is a highly specialized field, and individual doctors may offer different creative approaches. It is best to speak to a qualified specialist if you decide to go this route. By working with a chronic pain specialist, you may gain enough temporary relief to be able to step back and assess your situation more clearly. It is important to remember that IC is really a systemic disease, and you may never be entirely well until you determine what is causing or exacerbating your symptoms beyond your ability to manage them. Although I believe in investigating and treating IC and other painful chronic disorders in a holistic way, I would *never* advise anyone to go without adequate pain relief for any reason. Below, Bill shares his powerful success story with us:

CASE STUDY: *Bill's Success Story*

I've had IC for ten years. For eight of those years, I experienced daily pain, urinary urgency, stress, fear of food, and many food allergies. I was often up five or more times during the night. Of the many things I tried, Dr. Wise's workshop on treating chronic pelvic pain was most helpful, but pain inhibited my ability to fully utilize the stretching exercises I learned there.

Two years ago I had a breakthrough when a friend suggested I try a nerve block (epidural). This friend's mother receives two nerve blocks annually to relieve her pain. I underwent the maximum of three blocks over a six- to eight-month period. After the first one, my pain went from a ten to a six the next morning. After the second one, my pain was entirely gone! After a few months it began to come back, though not as acutely or as often as in the past. I've now been fine for eighteen months, and I don't anticipate needing another one. And I have the security of knowing I can return to the nerve block protocol if needed. This security has replaced the despair of too many years of chronic pain. My relief from pain also means a relief from the daily stress of anticipating and experiencing pain. To let go of years of daily physical and emotional pain is like night and day...a welcome return to quality living.

Now I void maybe twice during the night. I rarely experience pain, frequency, or urgency. During the day I can sometimes go for two or two-and-a-half hours without voiding, a big improvement. I can exercise as much as I want (strength training, aerobics, stretching), which is a great stress reducer, along with providing other benefits to my general health, well-being, and self-esteem. A surprising additional bonus was the resolution of more than twenty-five food allergies I developed as a result of IC, which I believe is an immunological disease.

When a nerve block was first suggested by my friend, based on her mother's experience, I assumed it would involve surgery or some sort of implant that would block *any* feeling traveling from the pelvic area to my brain, which could be dangerous. A year later I learned from my friend that it was simply an injection that would cause minor discomfort, lasting maybe two minutes. So I called a highly respected pain specialist for an evaluation. At that point I was wishing my IC would either get better or do me in, so when I was asked in the evaluation to state my pain level on a scale from zero to ten, I said, "How about thirteen?"

My doctor explained that the worst outcome would be that the procedure would have no effect—or, that it could work for a few hours, days, weeks, or months. Or, I might never need another one. Those sounded like good odds. Before my first procedure I wasn't informed that for a few hours following injection the pain might temporarily worsen. So when the pain did get worse, I felt hopeless. But when I woke up the next morning the pain had decreased significantly,

(cont'd.)

and it felt like a miracle. A couple of months later, with my second injection, I was ready for the short-term temporary increase in pain.

I wish I had known about this technique years before. The turning point in my journey to restore my life, happiness, and self-esteem was a painless two-minute nerve block. It might not work for everyone, but I'm hopeful that others with IC can receive total relief from chronic pain with a series of nerve blocks done by a pain specialist.

What You Can Do Now

You've now learned what allopathic medicine can offer you. Many of these options may appeal to you, and may, in fact, be useful to you at certain stages in your recovery. I encourage you to further investigate any specific treatments that seem appropriate to your situation and discuss them with your health practitioner. Still, I believe that the traditional allopathic or mainstream approach has been, at best, only moderately effective for far too long. One of the drawbacks to mainstream medicine is its intense focus on *temporary* treatment, most often relying on prescription medications. Many of my physician friends will say this is because it is what patients ask for — in fact, what they demand. This book takes a different approach — rather than focusing only on *treating* symptoms, you'll learn valuable information that may enable you to get at the heart of what is *causing* your symptoms. This is the key to long-term recovery.

The best thing you can do now is to prepare yourself to be open-minded as we explore a holistic approach to treating chronic pelvic pain — one that considers *every* aspect of your life and health, including self-care, food sensitivities, diet, stress, hormones, occult infections, and more. You can recover, step-by-step. Accept nothing less than a full recovery!

PART II

Beginning
the Journey

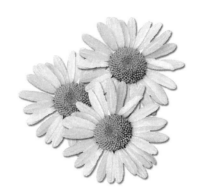

4

Learning to Manage Symptoms

The goals of this chapter are to teach you relaxation techniques; to help you embrace the importance of exercise; to share effective self-treatment strategies to alleviate pain, urgency, and frequency; to teach you how to improve your sleep patterns; to help you begin self-evaluation; and to teach you how to track your progress. All of these tools will assist you in managing your bladder symptoms on your way to total recovery.

Managing Stress

Let's start by addressing stress. The strategies presented in this chapter and those that follow are meant to begin dialing down pain and stress. This, in turn, helps to take the load off the overworked adrenal system, which controls our fight-or-flight response. Why do I say it is overworked? When we suffer from painful disorders like interstitial cystitis (IC) and chronic pelvic pain (CPP), our adrenal glands are continuously overburdened by pain, inflammation, and years of far too little sleep. The simple yet effective tools described in this chapter are designed to help you begin to feel better *immediately*, which in turn decreases adrenal stress. But before we can move forward, there's some baggage we need to leave behind.

Give Up Your Guilt

For those of us with any chronic health problem, it is important to move past the guilt we all sometimes feel. It can be very hard to sit back and let others do the things we want to be doing for ourselves and our families. Health problems can also have drastic financial consequences, especially if we must give up our jobs due to health circumstances or if we lack adequate health insurance. However, feeling guilty just adds to our stress burden and does nothing to move us along the path toward healing. It is necessary to forgive ourselves and say "goodbye" to guilt in order to begin healing. *We are ill through no fault of our own.* IC and CPP are not something we asked for or contributed to by abusing our bodies. Life happens — sometimes not in the way we want. We all do the best we can to adapt.

Learn to Relax

One of the keys to health is relaxation. Learning to relax is key to recovering from any chronic illness, but it is *essential* for anyone suffering from bladder symptoms or pelvic floor dysfunction. Trust me on this! You will learn much more in later chapters about why relaxation is so important. For now, let's try a couple of basic relaxation exercises, beginning with deep breathing.

Exercise **Deep Breathing**

Lie down or sit comfortably. Count slowly to four as you inhale through your nose, and count slowly to four as you exhale through your mouth. This technique is a good way to wind down at the end of the day, and I have often used it to help fall asleep. It usually only takes a few minutes. Practice this breathing exercise and see if it brings your pain level down a few notches. If you like, you can focus on a word or mantra that you associate with each phase of your breathing. A simple one is "Breathe in health, breathe out pain."

Exercise **Relaxing from the Toes Up**

This is a very simple technique I learned in nursing school. Lie down or sit comfortably, and close your eyes. Breathe deeply and try to relax; do a minute or two of the deep-breathing exercise. Then focus

(cont'd.)

on your toes, and consciously relax them. Repeat to yourself, "Relax my toes," and keep breathing calmly until the toes feel relaxed. Ever so slowly, move your way up the body, paying attention to each area in turn. Focusing on each area individually for the minute or so it takes to relax will help you become intimately familiar with the areas of the body where you hold the most tension—they will take longer to relax.

Benefits of Daily Exercise

We all know the benefits of exercise in improving and maintaining fitness and helping to prevent conditions such as high blood pressure, diabetes, and cardiovascular disease. But exercise does more than that; it provides very real benefits in reducing levels of stress and anxiety, helping our bodies deal with chronic pain, and enhancing our immune systems. If you take into account the natural vitamin D from sun exposure, and the benefits of exercise on chronic inflammation, going for a run or a brisk walk has a great deal to offer for overall health.

If you are suffering from sleeplessness, chronic pain, and bladder frequency and urgency, exercise might be the furthest thing from your mind. I hope that after reading more about it, you'll realize how important exercise is to your overall well-being and make it a goal to get at least some amount of exercise each day. Exercise can take many forms, and you can begin with baby steps. You may have heard the saying, "A journey begins with a single step." You may need to begin by walking around the block where you live. Don't discount any beginning attempts at exercise as trivial; you're making an effort, and when it comes to moving your body, every effort counts! This section outlines some of the many benefits of exercise and suggests moderate exercises that are perfect for people with IC.

Reducing Stress

I repeat—reducing stress is *essential* to recovering from chronic pain or chronic illness. Seven out of ten adults in the United States report experiencing stress or anxiety daily.[1] Those who suffer from chronic pelvic pain or IC have an added stress—one that never goes away, makes the activities of daily life more difficult, and interferes with restorative sleep. Activities that help us cope, such as talking with friends and family, and distracting entertainment, such as TV, movies, and listening to music, can be helpful, but other coping mechanisms, such as excessive eating or sleeping, can be harmful over time. One of the best ways to reduce stress, and the one most frequently recommended by health professionals, is regular exercise. Aerobic exercises such as walking, running, and swimming help to boost cardiovascular fitness as well. Low-impact exercises such as yoga, tai chi, and qigong (pronounced *chi-kung*) focus on breath and movements that release negative emotions. They can increase muscle tone, improve balance and coordination, and reduce stress.

How exercise helps to reduce stress and anxiety isn't entirely clear, but researchers generally agree that it improves mood, reduces anxiety, and helps people cope better with stress, perhaps especially physiological stresses such as chronic pain and illness.

The relaxing, stress-relieving effect of exercise lasts for less than a day.[2] This is another good reason to make regular exercise a part of your life. This doesn't mean that you need to take up marathon running tomorrow. Light to moderate exercises such as walking or swimming decrease anxiety as effectively as vigorous running. Recreational, skill-based activities such as golf or tennis also help to reduce stress. It is important to choose an exercise that suits your lifestyle, accommodates your current fitness level, and provides enough enjoyment for you to stick with it.

If your anxiety and stress are chronic, and anxious thoughts intrude frequently into your daily life, you may benefit from including meditation, positive imagery, prayer, or Eastern exercises such as yoga, tai chi, or qigong. Studies of practitioners of Asian-influenced martial arts like tai chi and qigong show that even simply going through the steps in your mind has measurable effects on stress reduction and the relaxation response. Surprisingly, I found this to be true when recovering from pelvic surgery. Even lying in my recliner, I could take myself to that inner place of relaxation — my breathing would deepen, my muscles would relax, and my pain would decrease significantly.

There are many good DVDs, websites, and books to choose from on these topics, but one of the best ways to participate is to take a class. This affords you the opportunity to meet others, get out of the house into a change of environment, and receive personal guidance on learning these ancient forms of meditative exercises whose positive health benefits have been known for thousands of years.

A few last words on stress: I live by the old Southern saying "Don't borrow trouble" — a quaint way of describing the bad habit of asking, "What if…?" I've learned instead to stay in the present and take one day at a time.

Relieving Pain

Exercise increases the release of endorphins, hormonelike substances that are the body's natural response to pain. In addition to boosting feelings of well-being, endorphins are known to have a pain-masking effect. Endorphins are produced during exercise and during periods of deep relaxation; they attach to the limbic and prefrontal areas of the brain, areas associated with emotions and mood.

Other studies have shown that exercise has a significant effect on pain perception and pain threshold. In one such study, the pain threshold (the amount of stimulus needed to elicit a pain response) was significantly higher and pain perception significantly lower in participants who cycled for thirty minutes than in the group who were sedentary.[3] Studies evaluating the effects of a tai chi regimen in the elderly showed improvements in flexibility, balance, pain, mood, range of motion, and anxiety.[4]

Endorphins are powerful medicine. Exercises that are most likely to result in endorphin release include moderate, continuous workouts such as running, swimming, cross-country skiing, cycling, rowing, and aerobics. Team sports such as basketball and soccer also fit the bill. It is recommended to do at least thirty minutes of moderate exercise every day, but cross-training, or alternating exercises, is always a good idea to prevent injury.

Boosting Immunity

In a study reported in *Sports Medicine,* moderate exercise was shown to provide immune-system protection.[5] In comparison with inactivity, frequent brisk walking reduced sick days by half over a twelve- to fifteen-week period.[6] Another study, of women athletes, showed that thirty-minute periods of regular moderate exercise increased circulating levels of immunoglobulins, which have a powerful protective effect on the immune system; levels remained high for up to several days, showing what a powerful and lasting effect exercise can have on the immune system.[7]

Reducing Inflammation

Low- to moderate-intensity exercise can help to decrease inflammation. Chronic systemic inflammation contributes to many age-related diseases, including heart disease, but it also plays an important role in many autoimmune diseases and in chronic pain. The regular muscle contractions of physical exercise help to release chemical messengers that suppress inflammation.[8] Exercise also increases the flow of lymph fluid and improves general circulation, which helps to move inflammation and toxicity out of the body.

In a study reported in 2004, two markers of chronic inflammation (c-reactive protein and tumor necrosis factor) were examined as they related to physical activity. The study concluded that the "inflammatory markers were lower in older adults with higher levels of exercise," but they were higher in the sedentary older adults.[9] Exercise really does help to keep inflammation in check—yet another reason to trade your slippers for sturdy walking shoes.

Alleviating Depression

In addition to masking pain and altering pain perception, endorphins can produce feelings of general well-being. Physically active people tend to be more resistant to depression, and to recover from it more quickly, than their sedentary counterparts.[10] In 2004 a review of studies documenting the effect of exercise on anxiety, depression, and mood confirmed the benefits of regular exercise programs. Subjects showed positive changes in feelings of anxiety and depression after even a *single* session of exercise.[11] Although endorphins are thought to be responsible for much of this effect, it is possible that increased circulation to the brain may affect the hypothalamic-pituitary-adrenal system (HPA axis), which controls physiological responses to stress. Exercise also increases other mood-boosting substances, including adrenaline and the neurotransmitters serotonin and dopamine.

Many of us know from experience that even ten to fifteen minutes of moderate aerobic exercise can leave us feeling refreshed and energized, more mentally alert, and better able to cope with stress or feelings of sadness and loss. When we take our exercise outdoors, we can breathe in fresh air, experience the sights and sounds of nature, absorb the sun's warmth, obtain vitamin D — the sunshine vitamin — and tune in to the seasonal rhythms of the earth. All of these elements can enhance the power of our bodies to heal.

There are so many benefits to regular exercise, and setting aside half an hour a day is all it takes. For those new to exercise, or those who are very ill, starting with ten to fifteen minutes of light exercise three days a week is a good beginning. You can increase your efforts as you gain strength and vitality. Adding a few minutes a day after the first week or so is often very achievable. It is a good idea to check with your physician before beginning a new exercise program, especially a strenuous one. However, almost anyone can begin with some light stretches, deep breathing, gentle yoga positions, or simply walking around the neighborhood. Exercise — it does a body good!

Tips and Tools
for Relief and Wellness

The following simple practices are designed to help you manage the pain, urinary frequency, inflammation, anxiety, and difficulty sleeping associated with bladder symptoms. They're based on personal experience and are backed up by sound science. Some will sound familiar, and some may be new to you. Take the first steps in gaining control over your bladder pain by following the strategies suggested below.

Stay Well-Hydrated

The human body needs a minimum of 1,500 ml of water a day to stay hydrated. That's a liter and a half, or roughly a quart and a half. If you are an athlete, exercise frequently, have increased metabolic needs, are ill, tend to perspire heavily, are taking antibiotics, or are detoxing, your body's need for water will be greater. If you suffer from constipation, you should drink at least an additional 500 ml of water. Our bodies are made of 75 percent water, and we simply feel better when we are well-hydrated.

The pH of water, or how acidic or alkaline it is, varies with the region of the country and the minerals the water contains, but in general water is neutral in pH compared to many other beverages, so it helps to neutralize any irritating substances in your urine.

Drink up! If you are worried about water intake increasing your frequency, you can take some precautions, such as sipping water throughout the day rather than drinking it in larger quantities, and you can cut back on liquids in the early evening hours, in preparation for bedtime.

Avoid Common Bladder Irritants

A recent study documented the profound effect of diet on bladder symptoms in IC. Of more than one hundred patients surveyed, 90 percent reported that eating certain foods or drinking certain beverages exacerbated their symptoms.[12] This study supports what those of us with IC have long known to be true.

You'll learn much more about food sensitivities and how they affect the bladder and other tissues in the next few chapters. For now, it is important to begin eliminating the most common food sources of bladder irritation. Many of these are "extreme foods" that contain acids, tannins, or high levels of salt, all of which can act as irritants to sensitive tissues in the same way that lemon juice might irritate a cut in your hand. High-oxalate foods are a special case, and you'll find more information on them in Chapter 13. Below is a list of foods commonly reported to cause bladder irritation in those with IC and overactive bladder:

- caffeine—espresso, coffee, tea, chocolate, green tea, soft drinks like colas and root beer
- vinegar—all types, but especially balsamic (for some people)
- alcohol—all forms
- soy sauce and other very salty foods

- sugar — white sugar, brown sugar, and other highly concentrated sugars
- tomato products — especially canned tomatoes (some people tolerate fresh tomatoes well if they don't overdo it)
- fruits and vegetables that are high in oxalates (oxalic acid) — including spinach, rhubarb, pumpkin, kale, and others
- citrus fruits and juices
- peanuts and peanut products
- yeast and fermented foods
- dairy products
- wheat
- gluten — contained in wheat, barley, and rye, and in foods made from these grains
- cranberries — despite helping to prevent urinary tract infections in people with healthy bladders, they can be quite irritating to people with IC
- chemical additives like MSG, potassium sorbate, sulfites, and aspartame, which have been reported to cause reactions in a great many people with IC

Sidebar   **Give Up Your Lattés and Frappuccinos**

A "perfect storm" of conditions caused by eating extreme foods (foods that are vinegary, salty, sweet, or spicy) and not drinking enough water will concentrate harmful substances in your urine and increase the likelihood of pain. Extreme foods include coffee.

Caffeine is one of the worst known bladder irritants! Coffee is bitter, acidic, and full of caffeine. It is a diuretic, which can increase frequency, and a stimulant, which can worsen urgency and trigger bladder spasms.[13] Simply stated, if you have bladder symptoms and continue to drink coffee (even decaffeinated), you will probably not regain your bladder health and will be contributing to your own discomfort.

One easy way to begin giving up your coffee drinks is to switch to "steamers," or drinks made primarily with steamed milk. You can request milk alternatives such as almond, rice, or hemp milk at many coffee shops, and add a very small amount of almond, hazelnut, or raspberry flavoring. If you're desperate for coffee, try a tablespoon or two of de-caf coffee in your steamer—just enough to give it a creamy color. (In Italy they call this a latte macchiato, or "stained milk," and it is sometimes given to children for a breakfast treat.) You can sweeten it with a little honey, agave syrup, or natural maple syrup. You'll still be getting a hot, foamy drink with depth and richness.

You coffee drinkers probably don't want to hear me recommending that you drink herbal tea instead, but I would highly suggest that you try a steaming cup of rooibos, or redbush, tea. It has a very hearty taste and a deep, rich reddish-brown color, it is naturally caffeine-free, and, best of all, it seems to be fairly safe for sensitive bladders. (Rooibos is often combined with other herbs in commercial teas, but for best results, look for straight rooibos tea.) You'll learn more about helpful herbal teas later in the chapter.

Neutralize Your Urine pH

Urine pH is a reflection of the body's pH, and the human body functions best when in a slightly alkaline (pH 7.3–7.4) state. This is best achieved by eating an alkaline and anti-inflammatory diet full of vegetables and fruits and lower in the heavy proteins, starches, and sugars that create acidic conditions in the body and lead to disease. Although there are a few acidic fruits and vegetables that are common bladder irritants, most fruits and vegetables are alkaline (see Chapter 6, "The Anti-Inflammatory Diet").

You may ask, "Well, don't the kidneys take care of balancing the pH?" Yes, they do. But the excess acid or base is secreted into the urine and ultimately ends up in the bladder. A urine pH of 5.5, the low end recorded by most urine pH strips, is extremely acidic; in some people such a condition can produce intense stinging, burning, and pain. This is especially true in someone with a bladder lining that is not completely intact, with a thinner, more fragile mucous layer, or with the pinpoint hemorrhages and ulcerations found in IC. Like lemon juice or vinegar on a cut, it is going to hurt!

Many people with IC feel as if their highly acidic urine is to blame for their pain and frequency, and certainly having urine more neutral in pH does help reduce pain symptoms, but it is more complicated than that. A 2008 study comparing inflammatory markers in the urine of people with ordinary urinary tract infection (UTI), IC, or detrusor muscle instability to those in the urine of healthy control subjects also measured urine pH. Patients with UTI had an average urine pH of 6.4; patients with IC had an average urine pH of 6.3; those with detrusor muscle instability had an average urine pH of 5.0; and those with no bladder symptoms had a urine pH of 5.5 (neutral pH is 7.0).[14] What this means is that a normal, healthy bladder is quite capable of handling low pH; it is the impaired bladder lining that makes low pH intolerable to IC patients. Raising urine pH to a more neutral level through diet and occasional use of baking soda in water is often helpful in alleviating symptoms.

Checking your urine pH is a good way to track your general health — whether your body is in an acidic, neutral, or alkaline state, and whether you are eating properly. You can track your progress over time. If you check your urine pH every morning for three to six months and keep track of the results, you will have a very tangible record of the progress you're making. In the beginning you may have a very low pH, but eventually you will hopefully be in the neutral range. At times, depending on what you've eaten or the medications you've taken, your pH may be slightly alkaline. If it becomes too alkaline, you may experience another type of burning discomfort.

Remember that drinking plain water, which is close to neutral in pH, helps to dilute and neutralize urine, potentially minimizing discomfort.

You can purchase inexpensive pH strips from a chemical supply store for about six dollars a roll. A roll can last for several months. You only need to tear off a two-inch strip each day. You can also purchase pH strips at a pharmacy or at an upscale natural-foods store. Make sure the pH range recorded on the strips ranges from about 5.5 to about 8, and that the strips are designed for human body fluids. The same strips can also be used to check saliva, another measure of your body's pH. "Hydrion" is perhaps the most common and reliable brand, and its products are available online at www.MicroEssential Lab.com.

Maintaining your urine at a pH as close to neutral (7) as possible may help you gain control over your IC. Many IC patients have long recognized the value of alkalinizing their urine through diet and the use of substances such as baking soda and calcium citrate.[15] A 2009 study documents that this approach really does help to alleviate symptoms, including nighttime voiding and sleep disturbances.[16] Patients in the study were able to raise their urine pH from 5.8 to 6.2. Patients who had more alkaline urine (at least 6.2) saw the greatest improvement in symptoms.

Calcium citrate can be obtained as an over-the-counter medication (Citracal is a popular brand). Its primary use has been to help prevent kidney stones, although whether it is effective for that purpose is controversial. Citrates were used in the study mentioned above on alkalinizing urine. Another option is using plain baking soda.

Mix ¼–½ teaspoon of baking soda in 8–12 ounces of water. Stir well and sip slowly. Its taste is not as terrible as you might expect, and it will be very soothing to your bladder. Drinking water alkalized with baking soda will help to neutralize the acids in your urine and raise the pH to a more comfortable and tolerable level. You can make this a regular practice if you don't suffer from high blood pressure.

This remedy seems to work so well for so many people that I can't help but wonder if it also has another effect. In addition to helping neutralize the acids in urine, one could hypothesize that buffering with sodium bicarbonate somehow helps to maintain the ionic charge associated with a properly functioning GAG (glycosaminoglycan) layer, although I don't know of any studies that support this idea.

Apply an External Castor Oil Pack

This was a very effective tool in bringing my pelvic inflammation under control. Inflammation in the pelvic cavity, in addition to the inflammation in the bladder lining itself, presses on the bladder, contributing to urinary urgency and frequency. I was a two-pads-a-day girl until I got my inflammation under control. I could not laugh, sneeze, bend over, run, or jump without experiencing some leakage of urine. It made me miserable. Now I can be active without wearing a pad at all! I really enjoy the feeling of freedom, and I feel more like my old self. Dietary changes had a great deal to do with decreasing my inflammation permanently, but regular use of castor oil packs helped, too, and they were also very soothing and comforting. This is a good treatment to use when you experience a bladder flare or accidentally eat gluten (assuming you're sensitive to it). Some people with chronic inflammation make it a practice to use castor oil packs three times per week.

Occasionally, castor oil pack treatments seem to disagree with IC patients. It may be best initially to try the treatment for a very short time until you know how your bladder will react.

To make a castor oil pack, fold an old cotton towel or piece of flannel into the size of the area needing treatment. Wring out the cloth so that it is thoroughly moistened with the castor oil (or simply pour castor oil onto the cloth). Place the oil-soaked cloth over your lower abdomen, and cover with a dry towel or plastic wrap. On top of that, place a heating pad turned to medium; turn the setting to low after the pack reaches desired warmth. Leave in place for thirty minutes to begin with, as the body can react negatively to the large amount of toxins initially drawn out of tissues into the lymph system and ultimately the urinary system. Wash your skin afterward with a mixture of warm water and baking soda. Keep the flannel pack wrapped in plastic and use as needed; discard after a few weeks.

Treatment can be applied every other day or only as needed. This is very helpful for inflammation and pain. You may void a large amount of urine after the treatment, so be sure to replace fluids and electrolytes. *If you experience leg cramps, weakness, lightheadedness, or any other adverse reaction afterward, this is not a good treatment for you.* Always use a high-quality, cold-pressed castor oil, preferably one that is hexane-free. Good varieties are available in health-food stores. Palma Christi is a reliable brand. *Note: Pregnant or nursing women should not use this treatment!*[17]

Seek Relief with Tiger Balm Patches

These inexpensive self-adhesive patches can be a lifesaver. They are small, portable, lightweight, and nongreasy. They do produce some odor, but it is not as noticeable as it is with Tiger Balm ointment, and most people find it to be pleasant. Tiger Balm Patches can be cut with scissors into halves or quarters, and they can be applied anywhere that hurts (on intact skin only). They work fairly quickly, within twenty minutes or so, to provide relief of pain that can last up to four or five hours.

One of the best uses for these handy patches is to treat the lower-back pain that is referred from the bladder. If you wake up after a tough night of bladder symptoms that include low-back pain, put a patch on and do a little light stretching, and you should feel better quickly. You can also apply a patch before you go to sleep, which may help you get to sleep by decreasing your pain level.

Tiger Balm's active ingredients include camphor, menthol, and capsicum extract, which work together to stimulate circulation to the affected area. When applied topically, these substances are also effective for short-term treatment of the pain of diabetic neuropathy, shingles, and fibromyalgia.[18] Capsicum is thought to help with pain relief by acting as a counterirritant, blocking the transmission of existing pain signals.[19] The patches may cause irritation if applied to freshly showered skin, but, otherwise, follow package directions and precautions for use.

Remember these three over-the-counter oldies but goodies — baking soda, castor oil, and Tiger Balm Patches — as potential pain-relieving remedies when you're fresh out of ideas or pain medications, experiencing a sudden flare, or travelling and without access to your doctor or usual medications. Any drug store or grocery store is likely to carry all of them, and together they add up to only about ten dollars!

Depend on Vitamin D for Chronic Pain, Including IC

Vitamin D has been touted in the news lately as a cure-all or preventive for everything from depression to cancer, and it is not just hype. As a species, we evolved to produce ample amounts of vitamin D when the sun's rays come in direct contact with our bare skin. With our modern, sedentary, indoor lifestyles, few of us get much sun, especially in the winter. This is particularly true of the elderly.

This isn't good news for our moods, our joints, or our bones. Vitamin-D deficiency, which is extremely common, can result in bone and muscle pain, and ongoing deficiency contributes to osteopenia and osteoporosis. This is because vitamin D is necessary for calcium absorption. It is easy enough to determine if a lack of vitamin D could be contributing to your pain and fatigue by having your vita-min-D level tested by your physician. If it is low, taking supplements and exposing your skin to at least fifteen minutes of direct sun a day (in the summer months) can help in a matter of weeks.

In a recent review of twenty-two clinical studies of patients with chronic fatigue and pain, researchers found numerous correlations with vitamin-D deficiency. The relationship was especially obvious in patients who had back pain. In one study alone, fully 93 percent of those who suffered from chronic musculoskeletal pain were mea-surably deficient in vitamin D, in some cases severely so. Vitamin-D supplementation was shown to cause chronic fatigue and pain symp-toms to disappear.[20] In a different study, reported in the *Journal of Internal Medicine,* a population of Danish women of Arab descent who presented with muscle pain and weakness similar to fibromyal-gia were tested for vitamin-D deficiency. Perhaps due to genetic fac-tors, 88 percent of them were severely vitamin-D deficient.[21] People with darker skin are thought to require more sun exposure to pro-duce vitamin D than do those with lighter skin.

Vitamin D, which is also sometimes called the "sunshine vita-min," is a fat-soluble, hormonelike substance. It is best absorbed in its vitamin-D-3 form, which is available as an affordable over-the-counter supplement. Vitamin D isn't naturally found in many foods, with the exception of fortified dairy products, some ocean fish, egg yolks, a few dark leafy greens, and cod liver oil. If you suffer from muscle aches and general body pain, fatigue, or depression, it would be wise to have your vitamin-D level checked, especially if your dis-comfort interferes with getting adequate, restful sleep. If you are se-verely deficient, your physician will order a larger temporary dose for you. In general, though, it is widely recommended to take at least 200–400 IU (international units) per day, and perhaps more in the low-light winter months.

Vitamin D plays an important role in reducing inflammation and, as an important immune modulator, may even play a role in preventing autoimmune disorders like multiple sclerosis and dia-betes.[22] Studies indicate that an epidemic of vitamin-D deficiency could also be linked to rising rates of cancers, including colon, breast, and especially prostate cancers.[23] However, some of the newest research on vitamin D actually pertains to IC. In 2006 a team of researchers in Milan, Italy, found that specific compounds of vitamin D-3 (not the kind you buy at the pharmacy) were effective in controlling inflammation in the bladder wall in allergen-induced chronic bladder inflammation, suggesting a possible new therapeutic avenue for treating IC patients.[24] Various vitamin-D compounds had significant effects on reducing inflammatory cytokines and on deactivating mast cells (which release histamine). Tissue examination of the mice used in the study backed up the findings with clinical evidence. This research was done using animal models, and much more work is necessary, but the results were promising enough for the researchers to secure a patent on a specific vitamin-D-3 compound, which is now under development. Stay tuned for more news on this possible new IC treatment!

How Brain Chemistry Influences the Body's Pain Response

Neurotransmitters can be thought of as chemical messengers that work together in a delicate balance. There are at least four neurotransmitters that transmit pain signals and four that inhibit pain. Those that are involved in transmitting pain are glutamate, substance P, norepinephrine (which can inhibit *or* enhance pain signals), and acetylcholine. On the inhibitory side are endorphins, the body's natural pain killers, which are released in response to pain signals and help to inhibit substance P and acetylcholine. (Remember, endorphins are also released when we exercise.) Another pain-inhibiting neurotransmitter is gamma-aminobutyric acid (GABA), which reduces the action of glutamate and substance P. Serotonin, perhaps the most familiar neurotransmitter, helps moderate pain in four ways—by helping to dull the brain's perception of pain, relaxing blood vessels, elevating mood, and producing a calm state (and, for some, inducing sleep). These are some of the physiological reasons why antidepressants that boost serotonin may be useful in the management of chronic pain.

The role of brain chemistry in chronic pain is very complex. Yet achieving this balance of naturally occurring neurotransmitters may be something the subconscious can control. This is one of the main theories behind the processes of visualization, positive visual imagery, and biofeedback. You can choose to work with a professional to learn these powerful techniques. You can also investigate use of the nutritional and herbal supplements discussed below, some of which target production of the neurotransmitters involved in the pain response.

Relieve Pain with Nutritional Supplements

Some nutritional supplements may be useful in managing pain and sleep. Remember, though, that it is important to avoid trying too many new supplements at once, and it is best to utilize the guidance of a skilled healer or naturopath, if possible. Here's another word of caution: The fragile IC bladder is very sensitive, and some nutritional supplements, just like some foods, are not well tolerated. So, if the directions say to take two capsules, take one. If they say to take one, then take half of one capsule. Another rule of thumb is to take capsules instead of tablets whenever possible. Capsules contain fewer extraneous ingredients that might irritate the bladder.

The following supplements may be helpful in alleviating inflammation and symptoms of bladder irritation and pain common in those with IC and/or pelvic pain.

Evening primrose oil, blackcurrant seed oil, and borage oil, which are all good sources of the essential fatty acid gamma-linolenic acid (GLA), are useful in reducing inflammation and have been shown to help in conditions of chronic pain.

DLPA (DL-phenylalanine), a form of the amino acid phenylalanine, has been used to help increase the pain threshold in chronic pain conditions. It does not occur naturally, but it can be found in supplement form. (Other forms of phenylalanine are naturally occurring and can be found in protein-rich foods.) DLPA seems to have some ability to enhance endorphins, the body's naturally occurring pain killers. DLPA may also boost GABA levels (see below).

GABA-boosting supplements, including 5-HTP (a serotonin precursor), methionine, and fish oils that contain EPA and DHA, may help with pain. GABA is the chief pain-inhibitory neurotransmitter in the human nervous system. It plays an important role in regulating nerve excitability throughout the nervous system, and it is directly responsible for the regulation of muscle tone. In the human body, GABA is synthesized from the amino acid glutamate and vitamin B-6. It moderates stress, anxiety, and pain, and it is thought to be deficient in some people who suffer from disorders that are characterized by these symptoms, especially chronic pain and fibromyalgia. Some of the symptoms associated with GABA deficiency are backache, headache, muscle tension, muscle twitches, anxiety, depression, mood disorders, and, interestingly, abnormal sense of smell. Cold hands, constipation, and allergies may also be associated.[25]

Fish oils offer the added benefit of helping to reduce inflammation. It is often recommended to take 3,000 mg of pharmaceutical-grade fish oil per day, but be aware that fish oil has blood-thinning effects and should not be used if you have a vitamin K deficiency or are expecting to undergo surgery. Other supplements such as vitamin B6, zinc, and manganese may play a supportive role in improving GABA levels. If you also suffer from fibromyalgia, it may be a good idea to add magnesium and malic acid to your regimen. However, taking supplements isn't the only way to address a GABA deficiency. Foods that help to restore GABA include almonds, bananas, broccoli, brown rice, lentils, and walnuts.[26] It is very important to know that some GABA-boosting supplements, including 5-HTP, may make you sleepy, so use caution before driving or operating machinery. It is a good idea to try 5-HTP at night, just before bedtime, when you have few responsibilities and can take advantage of its sleep-inducing relaxation. Some practitioners prefer to use the amino acid L-theanine, which may be more effective in crossing the blood-brain barrier than GABA itself, while providing the necessary elements to form GABA.[27]

Glucosamine sulfate has been suggested as a supplement that may help to rebuild the impaired GAG layer. Several sources recommend taking up to 500 mg, three times per day. It may take several weeks to begin having any effect.

L-arginine is an amino acid that has been suggested for use in IC, especially by Dr. Robert Moldwin in his book *The Interstitial Cystitis Survival Guide* (Moldwin).[28] Although a small study conducted by Yale University reported decreased lower abdominal pain, ure-thral/vaginal pain, and urinary frequency with the use of L-arginine, the Mayo Clinic has advised that most studies of L-arginine and IC show no improvement.[29] In addition, this amino acid supplement may have serious side effects, including increased risk of bleeding, increased blood sugar levels, and increased potassium levels.[30]

L-Glutamine, another amino acid, is perhaps a better choice for those with IC. L-glutamine is very important in maintaining a healthy im-mune system and in protein synthesis of the body's tissues, includ-ing mucosa. Specifically, L-glutamine is often recommended to help heal a "leaky gut" (a gut with increased permeability, which allows incompletely digested food proteins to pass through the gut wall—not a good thing). You will learn more about leaky gut in Chapter 13, but it is important to know that there may be an association between leaky gut and IC (which is essentially, a leaky bladder mucosa). L-glutamine has also been used therapeutically to treat those suffer-ing from inflammatory bowel disease and ulcers. This supplement is available as an over-the-counter medication in most health-food stores. Avoid overdosing, follow the manufacturer's instructions, and monitor your reaction closely. Negative reactions to L-glutamine are uncommon.[31]

MSM (methylsulfonylmethane), a form of the element sulfur, may have an anti-inflammatory effect on the body and help to alleviate pelvic inflammation in general, including bladder inflammation. This supplement, which is taken orally, may be a more acceptable regimen than having treatments of DMSO instilled into the bladder.

Medicinal herbs, including ginger, boswellia, turmeric, and pine bark (pycnogenol) have been shown to reduce inflammation associated with chronic pain conditions.[32] But by far my favorite herbs for the bladder are linden flower, ashwagandha (an Ayurvedic herb), and plain chamomile tea. (See also the sections on medicinal herbs in this chapter and in Appendix B.) There are many anecdotal reports of people controlling their symptoms, or even achieving remission, by making regular use of linden flower tea and ashwagandha in tea or capsule form, in particular. In my opinion, herbs are an economical and underused treatment for many chronic health conditions, and perhaps especially for IC. Many people with IC are very sensitive to medications, and herbs can offer an effective alternative with fewer side effects. It is important to work with a skilled herbalist when addressing serious health problems, but if you are not pregnant or nursing a child, you can try some of the milder, safer herbs listed in this chapter and in Appendix B, which is on medicinal herbs. Just be sure to let your doctor and your pharmacist know what you are taking, as *herbs can interact with medications or cause other health concerns.*

Fight Fatigue by Getting the Rest Your Body Needs

There is a great deal of overlap between chronic fatigue syndrome/fibromyalgia and IC. Fatigue is a natural response to the exhaustion that comes with frequent sleep interruption for those with nighttime urinary frequency. Fatigue may also develop in response to the demand of fighting a chronic infection, which places added stress on the adrenals, or due to a combination of causes including depression and chronic pain. It is also important to rule out anemia related to heavy menstrual periods or malabsorption of nutrients as a cause of fatigue; your practitioner can perform lab tests, including tests for iron, vitamin B-12, ferritin, hemoglobin, hematocrit, and red blood cells.

Natural sleep cycles are about three hours long. A lot happens in each of those uninterrupted three-hour-long periods that is necessary to restoring and repairing the body, and to organizing and storing information and memories. Do you remember the "brain fog" you experienced as a young parent with a newborn? That's what chronically impaired sleep can do to you. Impaired sleep can also lead to heightened pain sensitivity and other symptoms, including chronic fatigue and fibromyalgia (see the research highlighted on the next page).

To reduce muscle aches and pains, and to get better sleep in order to help your body to heal and enhance your ability to cope with pain, try to take whatever steps you can to facilitate restful and restorative sleep.

If you've been diagnosed with chronic fatigue syndrome and/or fibromyalgia, you may benefit from following an anticandida diet, described in Chapter 10, as there may be a connection (although the evidence isn't yet clear). Both chronic fatigue syndrome and fibromyalgia may have various causes, including viral illness, such as herpes virus 6 (HHV-6), perhaps in combination with Epstein-Barr virus (Yuan), which affects the immune system. And, recently, researchers identified a brand-new virus that may be associated with chronic fatigue syndrome. Interestingly, this virus, known as XMRV (which may also be associated with prostate cancer), was found in the blood of 68 percent of chronic fatigue patients but in less than 4 percent of healthy people.[33] Researchers affiliated with the study identified XMRV as a retrovirus, the same category of virus that causes HIV. (All retroviruses copy their genetic code into the DNA of the host in a specific way.) This means that any further antiviral research on XMRV is likely to benefit from the enormous amount of research done on HIV, which even now is beginning to bear fruit. Talk with your doctor about these possibilities, especially if fatigue is an ongoing problem for you.

Research | **Sleep Deprivation, Chronic Pain, and Fatigue**

I've mentioned fibromyalgia and chronic fatigue many times throughout this book. This is because these syndromes often occur together with disorders that affect the bladder, such as IC. In Mari Skelly and Helen Walker's insightful book *Alternative Treatments for Fibromyalgia and Chronic Fatigue Syndrome*, IC is listed as one of the common conditions that may accompany fibromyalgia and chronic fatigue syndrome. Likewise, many people with IC also complain of fibromyalgia and chronic fatigue symptoms.

In an early section of Skelly and Walker's book they discuss a remarkable 1975 study in which University of Toronto researchers were able to induce or create fibromyalgia symptoms in otherwise healthy students by interrupting their stage IV sleep! This is the type of deep sleep in which our bodies balance hormones and heal damaged tissues. Interestingly, Dr. Moldofsky, who conducted the study, did not need to provide much disruption to produce this effect; he simply played a noise at such a volume that the students didn't actually awaken, but were never able to deepen their sleep cycles to the healing, restorative stage IV sleep. Dr. Andrew Holman, who studies fibromyalgia, went so far as to state, "Fibromyalgia is the predictable consequence of stage IV sleep deprivation."[34] He believes this occurs in response to continually elevated levels of adrenaline from an overactivated stress response. Other symptoms of an overactivated stress response, in addition to elevated heart rate and blood pressure, include anxiety, muscle tension, and bowel and bladder tension. I find it interesting that once again the stress response is involved. Fortunately, this gives us an avenue to explore in terms of using stress reduction as a therapeutic tool.

Get a Good Night's Sleep

The studies discussed in the "Research" section above suggest to me that those with bladder problems that include nighttime frequency or "just enough" bladder tension or pain to keep the nervous system stimulated may also be suffering the effects of stage IV sleep deprivation. (It certainly feels like sleep deprivation!) The bottom line is that *getting adequate sleep is essential for those with chronic pain or chronic illness of any kind. It is how we heal.* Sleep also helps us cope with the pain we experience and with the challenges of daily life. Getting adequate sleep may require: first, treating pain; second, implementing stress-reduction strategies; and third, occasionally making use of medications or herbal remedies that assist us in falling asleep and staying asleep. Those with bladder spasms or pelvic floor tension may require additional medications such as muscle relaxants. Try to do whatever you can do to ensure you receive at least eight hours of restful slumber. The following is one simple strategy:

- Drink a cup of antispasmodic herbal tea after dinner, but not immediately before bedtime. Make sure you have enough time to void once or twice before going to bed. I suggest chamomile or linden, or a mixture of both. Also, see the list of recommended herbal teas in the next section.

- Before bedtime, take a warm bath enriched with Epsom salts, which contains magnesium and can soothe inflammatory conditions.

- During or after your bath, drink about ¾ cup of water, with ¼ teaspoon of baking soda stirred in, to help neutralize your urine.

- Take one or two capsules of ashwagandha for general relaxation or, if you have problems sleeping, about 100 mg of 5-HTP. (Always use the lowest dose of a supplement or medication, and try it on a night when you don't have to go anywhere or do anything the next day, until you know how you're going to react.)

- Dry your skin well, and place a Tiger Balm Patch over the area of your abdomen or pelvis that feels most uncomfortable. Tiger Balm Patches can be cut to size.

- You should make your sleeping space as relaxing and conducive to restful sleep as possible. Then, slip between clean, cozy sheets and do ten minutes of deep breathing or progressive relaxation from the toes up.

- If you happen to wake up at night and cannot get back to sleep, take GABA or melatonin as directed. If bladder spasms are waking you, try ashwagandha. You can also take skullcap, a much stronger herb with antispasmodic properties. Regular chamomile tea is also worth a try, as it is quite a good antispasmodic. Sweet dreams!

Drink Soothing Medicinal Teas and Herbs

Drinking medicinal teas can help us stay well-hydrated, neutralize and dilute our urine, and bring our bodies back into a slightly alkaline state for better health. It is a good idea to become familiar with the use of these traditional medicines, which can be both effective and economical. Learn to relax and take pleasure in a steaming cup of tea when you're feeling low on a chilly day. I've listed several categories of helpful herbs here, along with some specific tea blends that have brought me relief. (See Appendix B for more on herbs that soothe the bladder.)

For irritated tissues: Mucilaginous or "demulcent" herbs help to coat and soothe irritated, inflamed tissues; these include marshmallow root, linden flower, slippery elm, couch grass, and plantain.

For pain: Use birch leaf or white willow bark for moderate to severe pain; chamomile for mild discomfort. Goldenrod can be useful for back pain referred from the bladder or for arthritic back pain. Skullcap can be used in capsule form for nerve pain and as a general pain reliever, but it is quite sedating. Linden is a much-milder relaxing herb that I highly recommend.

For spasms: Use fennel seed, linden flower, skullcap (loose herb tea or an herbal capsule), chamomile (weakly brewed). One of the best is the Ayurvedic herb ashwagandha, available in capsules and tincture.

For inflammation: Use chamomile, marshmallow root, red raspberry leaf, slippery elm. Some other herbs that are good for inflammation are potent diuretics, and thus are not useful for those who suffer from urinary frequency. It is best to try such herbs earlier in the day and when you're at home near a bathroom (See Appendix B for more herbs to treat bladder symptoms.)

Sidebar — **My Personal Favorite Herb Blends**

The following are some combinations of herbs that have given me good results:

Nighttime Tea
It is best to drink this after dinner, but give yourself time to void at least once or twice before going to bed.

Equal parts linden flower, marshmallow root, and slippery elm. For flavor, brew with one chamomile tea bag or a little loose chamomile tea, if desired. If you continue to let the tea steep overnight, the mucilaginous properties of the marshmallow and slippery elm will develop, and the next morning you can dilute it and drink it to start your day pain-free. If you need a little help with sleep or have trouble with bladder spasms, add a pinch of pleasant-tasting skullcap or cat-mint (nepeta) to make you feel relaxed and drowsy, but be sure to avoid these two herbs during the day or any time when alertness is required, such as when driving.

Calming-a-Flare Tea
Equal parts linden flower, marshmallow root, plantain, birch leaf (or white willow bark), and wood betony (or skullcap). This is a combination of soothing demulcent herbs, anti-inflammatories, and pain

(cont'd.)

relievers. If you think your flare may be triggered by stress, drink tea with two capsules of ashwagandha to reduce anxiety, especially if you're having bladder spasms. If you feel there's an infectious component, add an additional equal amount of pipsissewa and arrange to see your doctor. If you feel food sensitivities are involved, consider adding a large pinch of nettle leaf and be as conscientious as possible about your diet.

It's-My-Period-and-I'll-Cry-If-I-Want-to Tea

Plain chamomile, with a *pinch* each of red raspberry and lemon balm. (Cramp bark is also very effective and it is often available in a tincture form. (See Appendix B for more on herbal remedies for the bladder.) If steeped too long, raspberry leaves can become very astringent and bitter, and the essential oils in lemon balm can become overwhelming. It is best to use only a small amount and steep for only a few minutes, until a pale-green color develops.

What You Can Do Now

Self-assessment is an important part of any recovery plan. In a journal, keep track of any changes you are beginning to make in your lifestyle (including relaxation), exercise, diet, and symptom management. Begin using self-soothing techniques such as castor oil packs, applications of warmth or cold, baking-soda water, etc.

Experiment with dietary supplements and herbal teas as desired. These small changes may give you greater control over your bladder symptoms and pelvic discomfort.

Improved sleep can yield welcome positive changes in your overall health, and, importantly, in your ability to handle pain and stress. Follow the sleep tips suggested in this chapter; do your best to lower stress, particularly in the evening, and try to get some deep, healing sleep. This is probably the most important thing you can do for your state of mind, your immune system, and your bladder, too.

The "Daily Bladder Diary," below, can be used every day to record your progress and allow you to see trends. You can easily use it as a guide to set up a spreadsheet or journal on your computer. In it, rate your pain, urinary frequency, and anxiety. Remember to also check and record your urine pH. If it is in the low range, less than 6.25, try drinking a glass of water with baking soda. Rate your pain level before and after, and record the results.

Daily Bladder Diary

On a scale of 0–10, with 10 being the worst pain, rate your pain level throughout the day:

morning _____　　　noon _____

dinner _____　　　bedtime _____

during the night _____

During these same time periods, count or estimate the number of times you voided:

morning _____　　　noon _____

dinner _____　　　bedtime _____

during the night _____

On a scale of 0–10, rate your anxiety level at the following times, whether or not you feel it is related to your bladder symptoms:

morning _____　　　noon _____

dinner _____　　　bedtime _____

during the night _____

Daily morning urine pH _____

5

What's Bugging Your Bladder? The Role of Food Sensitivity in IC

The goal of this chapter is to illustrate the link between food sensitivities and bladder symptoms. The connection is real and could be affecting you. Based on my review of the clinical literature and experience working with individual patients, I've learned that food sensitivities play a *huge* role in causing or worsening bladder symptoms in a large number of people. As you'll read in this chapter, food sensitivities can also contribute to harmful inflammation throughout the body.

It is well documented that a large number of people with IC and other bladder conditions report suffering from food allergies.[1] In 2006 an interesting case was reported in which a woman treated for anaphylaxis with Omalizumab, a drug used to treat severe asthma, showed a significant improvement in her intractable IC symptoms while on the drug. The study's authors postulated that IC might be an "IgE-mediated, mast-cell-driven allergic disorder" — one that affects the urogenital system in addition to causing other commonly reported allergic symptoms (rhinitis, asthma, hives, etc.).[2] As mentioned earlier, increased mast-cell activity and histamine release, which can be associated with an allergenic response, have been found in those with IC. Dr. Theoharides of Tufts University has studied the role of mast cells in the pathology of IC extensively and has helped to form our understanding of mast-cell involvement in inflammatory disorders.[3] (Mast cells release histamine as well as other inflammatory substances, which trigger inflammation in the presence of allergens.) Dr. Theoharides' extensive research supports the role of mast cells in IC inflammation, but what causes the cascade of mast-cell-driven inflammation to begin? More research is necessary to confirm exactly how what we eat can *trigger* bladder symptoms and how gluten sensitivity, *in particular*, may play an important role in the disease process of IC; until now, this element has been largely overlooked. I believe following this line of inquiry will eventually lead to recovery for a great many IC patients.

There is another theory worth mentioning, and it also involves how our bodies react to what we eat. In 2008 David Klumpp, PhD, and Charles Rudick published an important study in *Nature* on a theory popularly called the pepperoni-pizza hypothesis. The theory is based on the fact that nerves from the pelvic region—the bladder, colon, and prostate—are condensed into a narrow area of the spinal cord near the tailbone, where they respond to signals transmitted from nearby stimuli, transmitting pain that may be experienced in an adjacent location.[4]

Some previous models of IC were based on the belief that symptoms were triggered by inflammatory substances in the bladder and urine—such as histamine, IL-6, and substance P—that were produced after ingesting certain foods. Klumpp and Rudick proved that another contributing factor is the "cross talk" between the nerves that affect the pelvic organs. Using laboratory mice, they created a condition that mimicked IC, injected the anesthetic lidocaine into the bladder, and demonstrated that the pain subsided. Then came the breakthrough: They injected lidocaine into the colon, and the pain in the bladder also subsided. In fact, according to Dr. Klumpp, lidocaine reduced the pain just as effectively as if it had been injected into the bladder itself.[5]

If eating a piece of pepperoni pizza irritates the colon, an irritation that is also felt in the bladder, then perhaps this phenomenon is applicable to other food-related symptoms, making it even more important for IC patients to examine the role that food sensitivities may play in their bladder symptoms. The idea, as explained in Klumpp and Rudick's article, is that those with IC have bladder nerves that are continuously transmitting pain signals to the spinal cord, and when a specific food, like the example of pepperoni pizza, irritates the nearby colon, an additional pain signal is sent to the same area of the spinal cord, ratcheting up the pain level.

Dr. Klumpp sees further research in "nerve-fiber cross talk" (also known as the pepperoni-pizza hypothesis) as a possible avenue for new treatments, including patches and rectal suppositories that could be used to control pain in IC patients and even possibly in those with other types of chronic pelvic pain. More research is necessary; fortunately, many important NIH-funded studies are underway.

In my opinion, the pepperoni-pizza hypothesis lends credence to the idea that food sensitivities may be more important than previously thought in triggering the symptoms of IC and other forms of chronic pelvic pain, but there are other factors that trigger nervous-system hyperexcitability, and these other factors may also be treatable. The nervous system, the adrenal system, the musculoskeletal system, and, perhaps most importantly, the immune system may work in concert to produce the typical cluster of symptoms that affect those with IC. These systems sometimes respond to the foods we eat in ways that may seem surprising and unfamiliar.

Food Allergies, Sensitivities, and Intolerances: An Overview

Allergists, naturopaths, and other enlightened practitioners know that food sensitivities can cause a wide range of physical symptoms, and that they are extremely common. Literally millions of people in the United States suffer from food allergies and sensitivities. Nearly 90 percent of all food allergies, though, are reactions to a small group of common foods: cow's milk (dairy products), eggs, peanuts, wheat, soy, fish, shellfish, and tree nuts (almonds, walnuts, etc.). Labeling of these food allergens is now required in the United States on all packaged foods. Corn is also a common allergen, but isn't included in the top eight list.

In my experience, few medical professionals are aware that bladder symptoms, too, may be caused by food sensitivities or food allergies. It is curious that this is the case, since it is certain that at least some researchers have known about the link for quite a long time. A study published in 1987, "Food Sensitivity, the Kidney, and the Bladder," stated that bladder pain frequently responds to elimination diets.[6] A 1984 study confirmed the phenomenon of eosinophilic food-induced cystitis in a closely followed patient.[7] (Eosinophils are white blood cells produced in both the immune response and the allergic response.) More recently, food sensitivities have been linked to bladder symptoms in pediatric allergies and bed-wetting, and they have been implicated in a study of IC patients in Sweden.[8] Furthermore, the anecdotal evidence is overwhelming that food sensitivities are extremely common and can provoke bladder symptoms.

Options for determining if food allergies or sensitivities may be contributing to your chronic health issues range from having blood work done to detect the antibodies IgE (involved in immediate food reactions) and IgG (involved in delayed food reactions), to having noninvasive energy-based food-sensitivity tests performed by a skilled complementary practitioner, to eliminating the most likely suspects for two to four weeks to see if doing so affects your symptoms.

True food allergies used to be considered rare, but they have been increasing in recent years, partly based on better diagnosis, although this is not the sole reason for the rise in prevalence. (There are all sorts of theories about why food allergies are on the rise, but this book isn't the place to go into them.) It is important to know that a true food allergy involves the immune system and triggers the production of antibodies to that particular food. Food sensitivities or intolerances can be related to poor digestive health, or they can be part of one's genetic makeup, due to an inherited enzyme deficiency. Lactose intolerance, common in Asians and some other ethnic groups, is one example (see "Casein" on page 102).

Some of the foods most likely to contribute to health problems, including inflammation and bladder-related symptoms, are discussed here. Unfortunately, you can see at a glance that they are staples of the standard American diet.

Sugar

Thanks to popular books like *Sugar Blues* and *Lick the Sugar Habit*, most people know that sugar isn't good for them. Then why do we consume so much of it? Why is it present in everything from spaghetti sauce to salad dressing to canned vegetables? Eating too much sugar is bad for our bodies. I am a former pastry chef who suffered from severe hypoglycemia (low blood sugar), and as a nurse I have taught many classes on diabetes. Believe me, I know sugar. Sugar contributes to tooth decay, gum disease, hyperactivity, and insulin surges followed by blood-sugar crashes. Excessive sugar consumption can raise triglyceride levels, which can lead to an increase in heart disease and atherosclerosis. The authors of a 2006 Swedish study even found that frequent consumption of sugar and high-sugar foods could increase the risk of pancreatic cancer by raising blood-sugar levels, thereby increasing the body's need for insulin and decreasing insulin sensitivity.[9]

Sugar contributes to illness in so many ways, mostly because we consume far too much of it in far too concentrated a form. Humans evolved to consume a piece of fruit, at the peak of ripeness, while walking or otherwise getting exercise — out there in the plains of Eden. We could only eat what we could carry in the palm of our hands, like a fistful of berries, or a medium-sized apple, plum, or peach. Isn't it convenient the way fruit is sized? A small banana, an apple, a pear, an apricot, or a peach provides the perfect amount of natural sugar for a quick energy boost. Unfortunately, it seems most humans are born with a "sweet tooth," and the more sugar we consume the more we want to consume.

Sugar is thought to affect the bladder negatively by altering the urinary mucosa, creating a surface that bacteria can adhere to, contributing to urinary tract infections. A sugar binge may also spill sugar into the urine, even in people who are not diabetic. Where there is excess sugar, microorganisms love to grow, so a sugar binge is an invitation to illness, whether a seasonal virus or chronic disease.

Other than the sugar occurring in fruit, the only sugars I recommend consuming, in small infrequent quantities, are natural, less-refined sugars like those contained in honey, maple syrup, agave syrup, and rice syrup. One of the best alternative sweeteners for those with blood-sugar problems is agave syrup. It is low on the glycemic index, meaning it does not contribute to a large spike in blood sugar. Xylitol, a sugar alcohol originally derived from birch trees in Finland, but now made from a variety of sources, is another low-glycemic sugar with possible health benefits, including reducing tooth decay.

Stevia is a natural plant-based sweetener that comes in either powdered or liquid form. Some people use it with good results, while others dislike its slightly chemical taste. One of the best choices is to take advantage of the natural sweetness of fruits and fruit products like applesauce, apricot sauce, and prune purée, all of which can be used in baking.

Soy

Soy, the darling of the food industry in the 1970s, 1980s, and 1990s, has been studied in depth over the past three decades. Although soy at first was lauded for its inexpensive, vegetable-based protein, anti-cancer properties, and natural phytoestrogens, nutritionists' regard for soy in the past few years has done an about-face. Among other concerns, soy can have an inhibitory effect on the thyroid. It causes an allergic response in many individuals, which makes it a particularly poor choice for use as a food additive (which is extremely common) or in products made for infants and young children, whose immune systems are still developing. Consumption of soy can contribute to bloating, flatulence, and other gastrointestinal complaints.

Soy's phytoestrogens have been found in three separate studies to inhibit normal ovarian function in women who are premenopausal. This is because phytoestrogens compete for certain estrogen-receptor sites in the body, preventing the body's estrogen from being processed normally.[10] Although some practitioners have suggested that soy may be helpful in controlling menopausal symptoms for women who aren't producing enough estrogen, soy phytoestrogens can actually cause problems in premenopausal and perimenopausal women.

Both of these sets of symptoms — gastrointestinal bloating and interference with the body's natural estrogen balance — can contribute to bladder symptoms. Bloating can press on the bladder, increasing urinary urgency and frequency, and hormone imbalances can contribute to urethral and bladder discomfort in other ways (see

Chapter 8). More generally, as we've discussed, if you are sensitive or allergic to a common food allergen, such as soy, consuming it will trigger the release of histamine, which contributes to inflammation of the bladder lining.

Casein

Casein is the protein found in cow's milk. It is different from lactose, which is a sugar present in cow's milk, although many people are sensitive to or intolerant of both. Many people who are gluten intolerant are also casein intolerant. In addition, cow's milk was designed by nature to be consumed by the offspring of cows, and it is conspicuously different from human breast milk. Although a good source of calcium and protein, cow's milk can contribute to a host of ailments, from joint pain, to sinus infections, to irritable bowel complaints. Physicians who treat patients with frequent respiratory infections, ear infections, and sinus infections will often advise them to avoid dairy products. Unless you are pregnant, nursing, or suffer from a family history of osteoporosis, you should be able to safely eliminate dairy from your diet. Interestingly, some people who cannot tolerate milk from cows can tolerate products made from the milk of goats or sheep, at least occasionally.

Lactose intolerance, or an inability to tolerate the sugar component of milk, can be hereditary, but it also often occurs in those who are gluten intolerant. This is because gluten, a specific plant protein, can damage the part of the intestine that is responsible for producing the enzyme lactase, which is necessary for breaking down lactose, or milk sugar. Gluten can damage more than the intestine, though, as you'll see in the next sections. Gluten may be playing a much more important role in your bladder health than you're aware.

People with a variety of chronic inflammatory and autoimmune conditions often do better on a casein-/dairy-free diet. This includes some people with IC, but also those with MS, rheumatoid arthritis, and chronic sinusitis. Dairy is one of the top eight allergens, and it is definitely one of the foods worth considering eliminating from your diet. (Remember that allergic reactions trigger the release of histamine, a bladder irritant, and contribute to inflammation in the bladder lining.) Today, there are many more healthful substitutes available because the number of dairy-sensitive people is so large. In addition, all vegan foods are dairy-free.

Gluten Intolerance
and Celiac Disease

Gluten, the substance that makes pizza dough stretchy and gives breads their great texture, is a common term for several related proteins found in wheat and its close relatives. In people with gluten intolerance, proteins in wheat, spelt, kamut, faro (or farro, also called emmer), triticale, barley, and rye are toxic. Oats may or may not contain gluten, depending on their source, and even oats that don't contain gluten (certified gluten-free oats) can provoke symptoms in some gluten-intolerant people. Gluten intolerance is more common among people of northern European descent, but is increasing around the world as the cultivation of wheat and related grains has spread. Gluten sensitivity is only one end of a spectrum of gluten intolerance, of which celiac disease is the most familiar presentation.[11] Not treating gluten intolerance through a gluten-free diet can lead to the development of more severe disease, including intestinal cancers. *The only effective treatment for celiac disease or non-celiac gluten intolerance is permanent adherence to a gluten-free diet.*

Celiac disease (CD), which is also called gluten-sensitive enteropathy (GSE) or celiac sprue, is a genetically linked, autoimmune, multisystem disease in which the gastrointestinal tract is the primary site of injury. Because nutrient absorption takes place in the small intestine, the damage caused by celiac disease results in malabsorption of nutrients and so extends its effects to other parts of the body. In celiac disease, ingestion of gluten triggers an immune response that causes inflammation, specifically in the intestinal villi, tiny fingerlike projections of tissue that increase the surface area for nutrient absorption. Repeated ingestion of gluten over time breaks down these tissues. Eventually the intestinal mucosa is severely damaged to the point that food proteins can "leak" through the gut wall into the bloodstream, triggering a host of food allergies and sensitivities, pain, inflammation, and autoimmune disorders, as well as neurological and behavioral symptoms.

Scientists who study celiac disease, such as Dr. Peter Green of Columbia University, sometimes refer to this disease as the "great masquerader" for its ability to affect virtually any organ or system in the body and cause a wide variety of symptoms.[12] Symptoms caused by celiac disease can be related to malabsorption from the damaged small intestine, or can be due to the direct effects of inflammation on various body organs and systems. Any doctor who states that you aren't thin enough to possibly have celiac disease, or that your diarrhea isn't severe enough to indicate celiac disease, isn't up-to-date on the latest research.

Although in the past research has often focused on the malabsorption problems of celiac disease—particularly in children with failure to thrive, small stature, iron-deficiency anemia, and chronic diarrhea (referred to as "classic celiac disease")—inflammation occurs in other parts of the body, and it is this inflammation that is thought to be a major factor in symptom development and in related autoimmune disorders. Many autoimmune diseases and neurological disorders are beginning to be linked to celiac disease and to non-celiac gluten intolerance.[13]

Non-Celiac Gluten Intolerance

Not all cases of gluten sensitivity are celiac disease. If you have celiac disease, by definition, you are intolerant of gluten. But it is possible to have gluten intolerance and not have "classic" celiac disease, because non-celiac gluten intolerance (also known as "acquired" gluten intolerance) can manifest in other ways. Those with IBS (irritable bowel syndrome) who respond favorably to a gluten-free diet may be gluten intolerant or gluten sensitive.[14] In fact, it is commonly reported that up to one-third of patients with celiac disease have previously been improperly diagnosed as having IBS. Both celiac disease and non-celiac, or "acquired" gluten intolerance, may lead to the development of autoimmune diseases and other associated disorders, and both are triggered by exposure to gluten.

One explanation of the difference between celiac disease and non-celiac gluten intolerance comes from Cleo Libonati's book *Recognizing Celiac Disease*.[15] Simply put, celiac disease is "inherited gluten sensitivity," in which inflammation in the intestinal mucosa leads to hyperpermeability, which may result in systemic effects throughout the body. Celiac disease is by definition an autoimmune disorder—it is the immune system's abnormal response to gluten exposure that causes the inflammation in the intestinal mucosa.

In non-celiac (acquired) gluten sensitivity, any damage to the intestinal mucosa has the potential to result in hyperpermeability (also called leaky gut syndrome), which may then result in systemic effects throughout the body.

Some of the possible reasons for injury to the intestinal mucosa resulting in hyperpermeability include: infection with an abdominal parasite such as *Giardia lamblia*, a bout with an intestinal virus, frequent or inappropriate use of antibiotics, poor eating habits resulting in gut dysbiosis (or an upset in the natural balance of internal gut microorganisms), or candidiasis (yeast overgrowth). However, one of the most overlooked and common causes may be the extreme overuse of over-the-counter nonsteroidal anti-inflammatories (NSAIDs), like ibuprofen, aspirin, and naprosyn, as well as stronger prescription drugs. These medications are well known to cause erosion of the mucosa in the gastrointestinal tract. And many people tend to ignore label warnings and physician's advice to take these products with food and a full glass of water. Drugs such as Advil are not meant to be popped like M&Ms. For some people, frequently treating fairly benign muscle or joint pain with NSAIDS is the beginning of a vicious spiral and the development of serious illness. Instead, I highly recommend topical treatments like medicated patches, massage, heat, and ice, applied appropriately, as well as regular exercise and relaxation exercises to reduce tension. We need to return to methods that worked prior to the development of these not-so-harmless medications.

Gluten Sensitivity and the Bladder: A Special Case

We've looked at the problems caused by gluten sensitivity—both celiac disease and non-celiac gluten intolerance. The body's reaction to gluten frequently affects mucous membranes. The bladder is lined by a very specialized mucous membrane, and now evidence seems to be adding up that gluten can be a big problem for those with bladder symptoms.

As we discussed earlier, bladder problems run the gamut — extended bed-wetting in children, frequency and urgency in young adulthood, stress incontinence after childbirth and continuing into the senior years, frequency/urgency syndromes in all ages, and bladder spasms or problems urinating in older men. We've already touched on many of these topics, which require fairly routine treatment. However, a surprisingly large number of people suffer from more serious problems, including recurrent bladder infections and interstitial cystitis.

Could there be a common cause underlying many of these bladder problems? One possibility is food sensitivities that trigger either an allergic response, an autoimmune response, or both. As we've learned, patients with chronic bladder pain and urgency often have elevated levels of histamine and other inflammatory markers in their urine. These findings can indicate that a heightened immune response in reaction to environmental or food sensitivities or allergies may be responsible for bladder symptoms. Another clue is that some patients experience relief of symptoms when on IV fluids, when too ill to eat solid food, or when following an allergy-elimination diet. Food sensitivities have also been implicated in bed-wetting in children, due to irritation of the urinary tract. And studies have shown that once food allergens are eliminated, the bed-wetting problem often ceases to be an issue.[16]

In some people, chronic inflammation and accompanying irritation may indicate the existence of an autoimmune condition like celiac disease. CD and IC often occur together, as reported by participants in support groups for both diseases. These anecdotal stories may have inspired researchers to begin taking a closer look at a possible association between these disorders. I was extremely pleased to learn that one of the first clinical studies was recently conducted by Chris Smith, MD; Peter Lotze, MD; Chris Jayne, MD; David Goldfarb, MD; and Fred Emmite, RPh, through Texas Medical Center, Baylor College of Medicine, in Houston, Texas. The study looked for overlap in the genetic expression of patients with interstitial cystitis and a reaction to gluten (including celiac disease) in thirty-nine female patients with confirmed IC. Other factors examined in this study were vitamin D status, gut dysbiosis, omega-3 fatty acid ratios, and secondary nutrients that may be depleted.[17] Preliminary results indicate a strong association between celiac disease/gluten sensitivity and IC in *all* subjects studied, and continuing studies have so far shown promising results in the subset of patients placed on a strict gluten-free diet. Look for the published study under the names of the principal authors, Dr. Chris Jayne, MD; Fred Emmite, RPh; and Baylor College of Medicine Urology Fellow David Goldfarb, MD.

The gluten-sensitivity/bladder-sensitivity connection isn't well known. Until I discovered it myself by years of trial and error, I would not have believed it to be possible. Following my subsequent recovery from interstitial cystitis and other health problems, I immediately began to advocate a gluten-free diet for those with IC or other chronic inflammatory disorders through several IC support groups. In 2008 I wrote about my experiences in healing from interstitial cystitis and other health problems by switching to a gluten-free diet, and I published the article on a popular celiac-support website. I have learned that I am not alone in making this connection. In fact, the response I received was overwhelming. People wrote to me from all over the United States, Canada, and the United Kingdom. Moms wrote about their children's bed-wetting clearing up, young women wrote about recovering from frequent UTI (urinary tract infection), and older women wrote to say that they no longer suffered from stress incontinence! All of the people responding to my article discovered the same phenomenon that I had: Excluding wheat and other gluten-containing grains reduced or eliminated their bladder symptoms. Could avoiding gluten really be the answer for thousands of people who suffer daily from bladder pain, urgency, frequency, and incontinence, or from IC? This question warrants further investigation, as evidenced by the many personal comments I received, a few of which I've included below:

- *I did not have bladder irritation or infection, but I did have stress incontinence. I was told it was 'normal' for a sixty-year-old woman. When I went gluten-free five years ago, my incontinence disappeared.*

• *I suspected a connection. Celiac disease is in my family. I asked for testing, but they said I wasn't thin enough to be suffering from celiac disease. Finally, I went gluten-free on my own. This cleared up my constant UTIs, hives on my legs and lower abdomen, bleeding gums, and all the intestinal distress. It's been fifteen months now and I'm feeling better each day.*

• *I have had IC for over a decade. I have been on a gluten-free diet for more than six years, and that has been the only thing that has given me any relief. I no longer take any meds at all—I haven't even been to a doctor for IC in several years. I would definitely suggest that anyone with IC try a gluten-free diet. It definitely gave me my life back.*

• *My IC first appeared in 1995, and the long road to being diagnosed with celiac disease lasted nine more years. Finally, I'm beginning to heal.*

• *I have both IC and a wheat allergy, which I ignored. I was paying the price with the severe pain of IC. Absolutely nothing was working, and no doctor would hear of the two conditions being related. Several told me that diet would not solve anything. That was until my experience with dermatitis herpetiformis (a variant of celiac disease) forced me to be gluten-free. The same diet has also completely stopped the IC pain. It's nothing short of a miracle to have my life back.*

The body's response to gluten can cause mouth, lip, and tongue ulcers, esophagitis, and deterioration of the intestinal villi (which leads to malabsorption of nutrients). It can cause pain and inflammation in the ileocecal junction (the area where the small and large intestines join) and in the pelvic and abdominal regions of the body. Is it any wonder that it can also affect the mucosa lining the bladder? Doesn't it make sense that inflammation in the area surrounding the bladder can produce both urinary urgency and frequency?

A physician wrote to me recently, stating:

My wife suffered for years with severe, incapacitating interstitial cystitis. In 2003 she was diagnosed with celiac disease. Since beginning a gluten-free diet, her interstitial cystitis has pretty much disappeared. I looked through the literature and found little research, but as a clinician I find the anecdotal evidence to be impressive. Why not the blad-

der mucosa? Celiac disease seems to stimulate autoimmune reactions just about everywhere else.

Screening IC Patients for Celiac Disease—A Great Idea!

Many IC patients suffer from gastrointestinal symptoms such as gas, bloating, discomfort, and diarrhea. Although such symptoms are often diagnosed as irritable bowel syndrome (IBS), it is possible that at least some portion of people with a diagnosis of IBS are actually experiencing a reaction to eating wheat and other gluten-containing grains. (At least 5 percent of people with IBS have active celiac disease, and the number who develop active celiac disease later may be even higher.)[18] It seems reasonable that patients with IBS symptoms, as well as those with IC, and certainly patients with both IC and IBS, should be screened for celiac disease and for non-celiac gluten sensitivity.

As a nurse I'm familiar with many autoimmune disorders as well as celiac disease. I also know there is some overlap between gluten sensitivity or celiac disease and many autoimmune diseases, including Sjögren's syndrome, rheumatoid arthritis, and psoriasis. For example, among patients with psoriasis, approximately 16 percent test positive for antigliadin (referring to wheat) antibodies.[19] (This is one of the tests used to diagnose celiac disease.) Of those 16 percent, nearly 91 percent experienced great improvement or remission of their psoriasis symptoms after three months on a gluten-free diet. As you read in the quotes above, many people with IC feel better or even have their symptoms resolve on a gluten-free diet. We don't yet know what percentage of IC patients have an autoimmune reaction to gluten, a gluten sensitivity, or a wheat allergy (although the evidence in the Baylor study, mentioned previously, is very impressive and should lead to further research). However, IC patients could be easily screened for celiac disease or gluten sensitivity at the time of their diagnosis, and sensitive individuals could be encouraged to follow a gluten-free diet. Patients who test positive could potentially be helped to recover from chronic pain and urinary discomfort, urgency, frequency, and incontinence.

For those of you who are willing to take on the challenge of a strict gluten-free diet, be prepared to be amazed at all the positive impacts on your overall health. Your bladder may feel wonderful, but your dermatitis may also clear up, your fatigue may vanish, and the swelling in your ankles may be gone when you wake up one morning. Your moods may stabilize, and your foggy brain may not be related to medication use or lack of sleep after all, but to gluten-related neurological effects. To help you get started, Appendix A, "Getting Started on a Gluten-Free Diet," provides a wealth of practical advice.

Research | Testing for Celiac Disease and Gluten Intolerance

According to Columbia University's Dr. Peter Green, an expert on celiac disease, the only definitive standard for diagnosis of celiac disease is an intestinal biopsy.[20] Others, such as Dr. Thomas O'Bryan, propose that a strict gluten-free diet trial is a less invasive as well as less expensive test.[21] There are also blood tests specific for celiac disease, including IgA endomysial antibodies (EMA) and IgA tissue transglutaminase (IgA tTG), both of which reflect tissue damage. Some doctors also recommend IgG tissue transglutaminase and total IgA antibodies. Antigliadin antibodies (AGA), which reflect a heightened immune response to wheat, are very useful in the diagnosis of celiac disease, and a new blood test, "deamidated gliadin," is able to detect measurable antibodies at earlier stages of damage to the villi lining the small intestine. The Mayo Clinic has replaced its gliadin test with deamidated gliadin, and the current recommendation is to test for IgG and IgA for transglutaminase and IgG and IgA for deamidated gliadin. With an IgA tTG of >100 and a positive response to a gluten-free diet, many practitioners feel that an intestinal biopsy is not necessary to confirm celiac disease. Make sure your doctor's lab is up-to-date, and arrange to have these tests done *before* eliminating gluten, as they are antibody based. If you stop eating gluten, your body will eventually stop producing these antibodies.

NeuroScience, Inc. (www.neurorelief.com) has recently developed a saliva panel that measures IgA and IgM for transglutaminase and IgA and IgM for deamidated gliadin and suggests that this test now has a sensitivity and specificity of over 90 percent. However, it would probably not be reliable for those with selective IgA deficiency. In addition, a test has been developed to detect celiac disease antibodies from stool. (A stool test kit can be ordered from Enterolab; www.enterolab.com). Ask your practitioner whether these tests are available and whether they would recommend having them done. Remember, *no test is 100 percent reliable in every person*; the very best test is a gluten-free diet trial for a minimum of three to six weeks, and a gluten-free diet trial is one of the *best* ways, other than the stool test, to diagnose gluten intolerance.

The Lectin Connection

Scientists always want to verify the "mechanism of injury." In this case, *how* does something like gluten, or the body's response to gluten, or perhaps other proteins present in gluten-containing grains, cause damage to the bladder lining and other symptoms? My theory stems from all the research I have read, combined with some scientific intuition. It seems likely that substances called lectins could play a role in the disease process of IC. Lectins are specialized proteins present in large amounts in grains, seeds, nuts, and legumes (and in some other foods). Wheat germ agglutinin (WGA) and the gluten components glutenin and gliadin are all potentially harmful lectins found in wheat. We now also know that WGA can directly damage tissues in the human body, even in those *without* a genetic susceptibility to celiac disease.[22]

Not all lectins are bad. Some are even beneficial. But for certain lectin-sensitive people, these proteins have the ability to elicit an immune reaction and cause a variety of negative responses. Many researchers believe that lectins are linked to autoimmune and inflammatory disorders, including rheumatoid arthritis and fibromyalgia.

Lectins are designed to withstand the hydrochloric acid in our stomachs and the action of protein-digesting enzymes. Like many proteins, some lectins may be destroyed in the cooking process, but many others are resistant to destruction by heat, especially dry heat, as in baking. The specific lectins found in WGA appear to be very heat resistant.[23]

How do lectins cause problems? They are involved in a process known as agglutination, or "clumping." (They are sometimes referred to as "agglutinins" or "hema-agglutinins.") The process of agglutination is actually an important mechanism by which the immune system latches on to invading organisms and clumps them together for escort out of the body. But some food lectins have the ability to agglutinate, or clump together, the body's own blood cells. This is because lectins have the ability to bind to certain kinds of sugars, including sugars we've ingested, but also the sugars that naturally make up cell membranes in the intestinal system and other tissues in the body. And because lectins can also attach to free-floating molecules, they can be transported throughout the body, causing systemic effects.

If you have a genetic tendency to react negatively to the lectins found in wheat and other gluten-containing grains, ingesting them can create a clumping of the blood cells in a particular organ or tissue. These clumps of cells are perceived by the immune system as invaders, and an immune reaction occurs, ultimately resulting in their destruction. Unfortunately, it doesn't take much lectin protein to clump together large numbers of cells in this destructive process.

Lectins have a special affinity for carbohydrate-rich or sugar-rich tissues, including mucosa, where they bind to the carbohydrate molecules that make up cell walls. Through their action, lectins can increase epithelial permeability and provoke an immune response that produces localized inflammation, as well as generalized inflammation in other tissues of the body. Some researchers believe this process may be responsible for causing the symptoms of irritable bowel syndrome and other chronic disorders; I believe this process could be involved in many cases of IC, particularly in those related to food sensitivities. It appears that powerful lectins binding to the carbohydrate-rich surface of the bladder mucosa may be responsible for a breakdown in the stability of this protective barrier, leading to an increase in the permeability of bladder epithelium, just as occurs with lectins and intestinal epithelium. Furthermore, lectins have the ability to stimulate mast cells to release histamine, which triggers inflammation in the body's allergenic response.[24] Research on food lectins only began in earnest in the late 1970s, and much more work remains to be done.

Focusing on the relationship between IC and the lectins in gluten grains yields intriguing possibilities. There appears to be a strong anecdotal association between celiac disease and IC, and also between IBS and IC. And, of course, there is ample anecdotal and clinical evidence that complete elimination of gluten grains from the diet can lead to a resolution of IC symptoms. I believe this is a promising line of inquiry, and I would urge researchers to study closely the association between gluten grains and chronic inflammatory diseases like IC.

What makes some people more lectin sensitive than others? Some people may have a deficiency of secretory immunoglobulin A, known as SIgA, a particular type of immunoglobulin protein. SIgA represents the body's first line of defense against foreign invaders, whether they are pathogenic microorganisms or protein antigens capable of causing an allergic reaction. SIgA is found in body fluids such as tears, saliva, and mucous, and in large amounts in human breast milk. Low SIgA is one of the factors that make people susceptible to lectin reactions and food allergies, and it may be one of the factors that make certain people susceptible to IC as well. What's really interesting is the relationship between stress and SIgA. The effect of stress on the body tends to temporarily *decrease* SIgA, which in turn *increases* the likelihood of food and environmental allergies.[25] This is because a deficiency of SIgA in the mucosa lining the intestines means that food antigens are not stopped at the "point of entry." Studies have shown that food-allergic individuals tend to have very low levels of SIgA.[26]

Another factor influencing lectin sensitivity is intestinal permeability. In general, anything that can lead to increased gut permeability, or leaky gut, allows greater numbers of lectins to enter the body's circulatory system, leading to increased lectin sensitivity.

The scientist in me wants to have the mechanism of injury verified, but the healer in me just wants people to stop suffering. Avoiding dietary gluten and other potentially harmful lectins can help at least some folks with IC. Other than waiting for science to catch up, can anything be done? Appendix A contains a detailed outline for going gluten-free. There are some additional suggestions you can implement right away, under "What You Can Do Now," at the conclusion of this chapter.

Recovery on a Gluten-Free Diet

My own health has improved tremendously on a gluten-free diet, but readers may wonder if there's a downside to excluding gluten. The negative that comes to mind is that such a diet requires more planning, especially in the beginning. It is also true that following a gluten-free diet can be more expensive, especially if you rely on ready-made gluten-free products. However, eating gluten-containing grains isn't necessary from a nutritional perspective—cultures around the world have thrived for thousands of years without them, and alternative grains contain many of the same nutrients, including protein, fiber, B vitamins, and the minerals iron, magnesium, and zinc. A gluten-free diet is based on the same principles as any healthy diet: It should include a variety of fresh vegetables, fruits, alternative whole grains, protein sources, and healthy fats. Brown rice, wild rice, corn, buckwheat, and quinoa are easy substitutes for gluten-containing grains such as wheat, barley, and rye. Less familiar nongluten grains include sorghum, teff, and amaranth, which are staples in Africa and Latin America. Your local natural-foods grocery store is a great source of these items, sold as whole grains or flours.

One of the questions I often hear is, "How long does it take for bladder symptoms to improve on a gluten-free diet?" This depends on how severe the problem is, and how long it has persisted. Some people actually begin to feel better in a matter of a few days, but others may take a month or more. Complete healing may even take several years in adults, although recovery is often more rapid in children. The good news is that trying out a gluten-free diet is relatively easy, and there is a wealth of gluten-free resources available to the consumer. If you feel better on a three-week trial of a gluten-free diet, then hopefully it is the answer you've been looking for.

I know that eliminating gluten may sound like an impossible challenge, so give yourself some time to think about it and to come up with a new plan for your diet. It is important to remember that simply by eliminating gluten, dairy, soy, and especially sugar, you are eliminating some of the most acid-producing, allergenic, and inflammatory foods in your diet, and you should begin to feel better *immediately*. However, it probably isn't a good idea to eliminate all of these foods all at once. Start by finding more healthful substitutes for the foods you already consume. For example, substitute a gluten-free bread, dairy-free beverage, or natural sugar source for your wheat, dairy, and sugar products. Learn to read labels. If it is necessary to take your reading glasses to the store with you, then that's what it takes.

Once you are comfortable with these steps, it is time to look more seriously at your diet, by starting either an allergy elimination diet (discussed in detail in Chapter 13) or another diet tailored specifically to your needs. I bring the allergy elimination diet up for a reason. Because both casein and gluten can damage the gut, people with gluten and/or casein intolerance often develop multiple food allergies. The foods that they ate while they were ill, before they eliminated gluten from their diet and began to heal, were not thoroughly digested before proteins from these foods leaked through the damaged gut wall into the bloodstream; in response, the body produced antibodies to these proteins. It will take time for the production of these antibodies to fall off, and that will *only* happen if the offending foods are eliminated until the gut has fully healed. Even then, some of these foods will continue to provoke a negative reaction.

If you have gluten intolerance, it will be a waste of time and energy to follow any specific diet until you completely eliminate gluten and begin to heal your gut. Your body will simply produce antibodies to the new foods you introduce into your diet as substitutes for those to which you were reacting.

Be sure to let your doctor know if you are sensitive to gluten, especially because gluten sensitivity has implications for autoimmune diseases, intestinal health, and even neurological and mental-health issues. Celiac disease increases the risk of developing diabetes and colorectal cancer, so gluten-sensitive individuals should be screened for these disorders. Men with urological issues or chronic pelvic pain should always be screened by their doctor for enlargement of the prostate and for prostate cancer. For more information, see the following websites:

www.celiac.com
www.glutenfreechoice.com

CASE STUDY: *Amy's Success Story*

I have had a lifelong struggle with my bladder and kidneys. Not too long ago I was in so much pain I felt like giving up on life. Now, after

(cont'd.)

a few weeks on a gluten-free diet, I feel amazing! I cannot wait to see how much better I will feel in the future. My son's diagnosis with celiac disease literally saved my life. I want to help get the word out about gluten.

I was so sick I thought for sure that I was going to die, and one of my family members was literally preparing to donate a kidney to me. It was also humiliating to go to the emergency room when I just could not take the pain anymore and be told, "Maybe you have a bladder infection," with rolled eyes. I actually once had a person from the psychiatric department talk to me about my "problems." They told me that I may have a mental condition or anxiety that was causing me to "overreact to my possible symptoms." People were losing faith in me fast. When I had a job, I frequently had to call in sick and therefore could not get a promotion. I was just stuck, a difficult place to be for an overachiever.

Going gluten-free ended all of this. I am so energetic! No pain, headaches, bladder symptoms—nothing! Before, I ate bread and instantly got a headache. I am amazed this was never suggested to me. I now feel like a thirty-one-year-old is supposed to feel. And I am *not* the drama queen everyone thought I was.

If you read only this chapter of the book, I will have done my job, which is to highlight the very real connection between gluten sensitivity and urinary tract symptoms. Other food sensitivities may also play an important role, but wheat and other gluten grains appear to be among the biggest offenders — not surprisingly, since they comprise such a large part of the standard American diet. If the gluten-free diet appears to have benefits for you, look for more information in Resources and in Appendix A.

What You Can Do Now

Consider excluding from your diet the following four foods: sugar, soy, casein, and, especially, gluten.

Eat a wide variety of healthful foods. Those who are acutely ill should eat primarily cooked fruits and vegetables, as they are easier to digest and less likely to produce antibodies than raw foods.

If you suffer from IC, ask your health practitioner to test you for celiac disease, using the recommendations presented in this chapter. If your result is negative, remember that you could still be suffering from non-celiac gluten intolerance. The very best test is a gluten-free trial diet, which means you would need to avoid eating anything made from the gluten-containing grains wheat, barley, rye, spelt, and kamut for a trial period of three to six weeks. Track your symptoms to determine if there is any change, keeping in mind that a complete recovery will take much longer. Be aware that other potentially harmful lectins include those found in corn, soy, peanuts, dairy products, and some vegetables in the nightshade family (eggplant, peppers, tomatoes, potatoes, and tomatillos).

Soak all beans and grains overnight, then discard the water and add fresh water before cooking. This helps to decrease the number of lectins in these foods and increases their digestibility for many people. Some people also soak nuts overnight, discard the water, then oven-roast them at a low temperature. In addition to diminishing lectin content, this practice can minimize reactions to mold in nuts, which are common. Sprouting of grains and legumes is very effective in minimizing the harmful effects of dietary lectins.

Consider taking a "lectin blocker," available from some online resources or through your naturopathic physician. Certain plants and nutritional supplements contain sugars capable of binding lectins so they cannot attach to the body's tissues and cause damage. Seaweeds such as bladderwrack (*Fucus vesiculosus*), and supplements such as N-acetylglucosamine (NAG), larch arabinogalactan, and slippery elm (*Ulmus fulva*) are often used to help minimize reactions to foods in lectin-sensitive people. They need to be taken prior to a meal to be effective.

Gaining control of your food sensitivities may help your digestion feel better and increase your energy, and you may experience a reduction in some of your symptoms. If you are feeling better overall, but you still have bladder symptoms, that annoying rash on your upper arms, or a runny nose and frequent headaches, it might be a good time to try an allergy elimination diet, described in Chapter 13, "Other Helpful Diets to Consider."

6

The Anti-Inflammatory Diet

We've talked a lot about food sensitivities and intolerances and how they affect the bladder. We've listed the foods that most commonly act as bladder irritants. But we're left with an important question: What is the best general diet to follow if you have interstitial cystitis (IC) and/or chronic pelvic pain (CPP)? Most physicians would recommend following some variation of the anti-inflammatory diet. This is relatively easy to do, and it is a good diet to follow for the rest of your life.

A Diet for Health

Because so many disease conditions, including interstitial cystitis and other causes of chronic pelvic pain, ultimately involve runaway inflammation, eating for health and recovery ideally means following an anti-inflammatory diet. Symptoms of urinary urgency, frequency, hesitancy, and stress incontinence will often subside once inflammation is no longer an overwhelming problem. Keeping the proper ratio of essential fatty acids in your diet is also very important when trying to treat inflammation. The typical American diet contains a far greater percentage of inflammatory omega-6 fats than is healthy. Omega-3 fatty acids, present in seafood, flaxseed, and certain oils and supplements, are very helpful in bringing this ratio back into balance.

Inflammation is prominent in the news these days, especially since recent research has linked chronic inflammation to cardiovascular disease. Inflammation is also a culprit in autoimmune disorders. Learning which foods, spices, and other substances help to promote or alleviate inflammation will give you a powerful tool for gaining control over your health.

Inflammatory foods tend to be "extreme foods" — foods such as vinegar, sugar, salt, alcohol, and cayenne pepper. But inflammatory foods also include those containing concentrated animal protein, such as eggs, red meat, and shellfish, plus many legumes and processed grains.

In contrast, anti-inflammatory foods tend to contain more water, are less concentrated, and include most vegetables, fruits, freshwater and ocean fish (especially those high in omega-3 oils), some seeds and nuts, and certain herbs and spices. Turmeric, the spice that gives curry its bright-yellow color, is a powerful anti-inflammatory common in Asian and Indian foods. Anti-inflammatory foods also tend to be more alkaline (that is, less acidic).

It isn't necessary to *completely* eliminate inflammatory foods from what you eat. However, it is important to be aware that your diet will affect you and to moderate it by making sure that the majority of the food you consume is alkaline and anti-inflammatory.

Some health advocates advise following an 80/20 rule: 80 percent alkaline and anti-inflammatory foods, 20 percent foods that may be more acidic in nature, like proteins or starches, and avoiding most or all "extreme" foods. This means filling up your plate with vegetables and salads, and including only a small portion of highly concentrated protein or grains. Note that this is a far cry from some popular weight-loss diets which advocate large amounts of animal protein. Some of you may have read Michael Pollan's book *In Defense of Food: An Eater's Manifesto*, the main point of which boils down to "Eat food, not too much, mostly plants."[1] It is also very important to always select the freshest locally grown produce you can afford. It is better for the environment, better for the people who produce it, and better for you and your family. Just like Mom used to say, "Eat your vegetables." It is still, and always will be, good advice.

Anti-Inflammatory Foods to Include

Choose freely from the foods on this list, or use it as the basis for beginning an allergy elimination diet. Note that with the exception of tree nuts, the anti-inflammatory diet does not contain many common food allergens.

Fruits: Unsweetened fruit and a small amount of fruit juice; choose from apples, pears, apricots, cherries, blueberries, peaches, raspberries, strawberries, watermelon, papaya, mango, and persimmons. You may not be able to tolerate all of these until your bladder is fully healed.

Vegetables: Raw, steamed, or oven-roasted vegetables; choose from green beans, zucchini, winter squash, broccoli, cauliflower, bok choy, artichokes, yams, sweet potatoes, cucumbers, celery, carrots, lettuce and other fresh greens and herbs, jicama, brussels sprouts, water chestnuts, and Jerusalem artichokes. Avoid only those vegetables that seem to be problematic for you *individually*; for example, some people are sensitive to vegetables that are very high in oxalates (kale, beets and beet-greens, spinach, and rhubarb; see Chapter 13) and many people react negatively to vegetables in the nightshade family (see "Inflammatory Foods to Avoid," below).

Grains: Brown rice and other forms of rice, millet, amaranth, teff, buckwheat, wild rice, quinoa, and other grains in small portions; small amounts of bread and pasta products made from nongluten grains.

Protein: Halibut, salmon, trout, sole, cod, turkey, chicken, wild game, lamb, and grass-fed (not grain-fed) beef. Remember to purchase sustainably harvested fish and humanely raised meat and poultry, if available. All seafood must be as fresh as possible or frozen to avoid the high histamine levels released as seafood ages and begins to break down.

Nuts, seeds, and oils: Cold-pressed olive oil, flaxseed oil, safflower oil, sunflower oil, pumpkin seed oil, walnuts, pumpkin seeds, almonds, sesame seeds and oil, tahini (sesame seed paste), almond butter, coconut oil, and unsweetened coconut.

Beverages: Unsweetened rice, almond, or hemp milk; spring water; most herbal teas; highly diluted, freshly squeezed fruit and vegetable juices.

Seasonings: Dill, oregano, cilantro, rosemary, thyme, turmeric, coriander, sea salt, and kelp. Stick with herbs, fresh or dried, for flavoring most foods; they tend to be milder than spices. Ginger is a good choice, if tolerated, because it possesses anti-inflammatory properties. Fresh garlic is often problematic for the IC bladder, but a little dried granulated garlic may be tolerated. Some people tolerate cinnamon just fine, while it seems to bother other people with bladder sensitivity.

Sweeteners: The healthiest choices are agave syrup, stevia, and brown-rice syrup; better still are applesauce and other fruit purees. Many people with bladder sensitivity find they cannot tolerate artificial sweeteners containing aspartame. However, xylitol, a sugar alcohol with health benefits, may be one lower-glycemic possibility to try.

Inflammatory Foods to Avoid

Below is a list of potentially inflammatory foods. Avoid them as much as possible, or observe caution when you do use them.

Fruits: Citrus fruits (lemons and limes may be used in small amounts, for seasoning, by those who are partially healed), dried fruits (especially those containing sulfur dioxide to preserve color), and grapes. There may be additional fruits that bother some individuals despite being both alkaline and anti-inflammatory.

Vegetables: Potatoes, eggplant, red and green peppers, tomatoes, and hot peppers. Avoiding these foods may be especially important if you have arthritis or joint pain and inflammation. Fresh tomatoes appear to be better tolerated than cooked tomatoes.

Grains: Gluten-containing grains, including wheat, barley, and rye. Oats may be tolerated by some people.

Animal protein sources: Grain-fed beef and pork; processed meats like bacon, salami, baloney, cured hams, and luncheon meats (some of these may also contain gluten); shellfish; eggs. (Some people may be able to tolerate eggs used in baked goods, but if not, use egg substitutes for baking. If you are sensitive to chicken eggs, you can substitute duck eggs.)

Nuts: Peanuts and peanut butter. Avoid any other nuts that are dark, discolored, or have a rancid odor.

Legumes: Dried beans, peas, and lentils, except in small amounts. Those with a sensitivity to oxalates must be especially careful.

Dairy products and fats: All milk, cream, yogurt, cheese, and other products made from cow's milk. Also avoid butter, all margarine and spreads that contain trans fats, and most processed oils, especially those that are heat-processed.

Beverages: Soda, black tea, coffee, alcohol, citrus juice.

Spices: Cayenne, paprika, black pepper, and other hot peppers.

Sweeteners: Refined sugars, including white and brown cane sugar, and corn sweeteners, especially high-fructose corn syrup.

Getting Started

As you can see, the list of anti-inflammatory foods far outnumbers the list of inflammatory foods, but the standard American diet (SAD) does contain a large number of inflammatory foods. It is no wonder that chronic inflammatory diseases are on the rise in the United States. Burgers, fries, milk shakes, sodas, baked goods, and cookies all have a negative impact on health, unless healthful substitutions are made. Here are a few suggestions: Substitute turkey burgers for beef. Skip the bun, or use a good gluten-free bread (no, that isn't an oxymoron). Make fries in the oven with white-flesh sweet potatoes and sea salt. Make a fruit smoothie instead of a milk shake. Add a salad to every meal, and create your own healthier versions of baked goods and cookies. Try to remember that concentrated sweets should be reserved for special occasions—not consumed on a daily basis. Your body will thank you. Please believe me about this, even if it takes some time for you to notice the difference. Your skin will be clearer and smoother, your stomach less bloated, your joints less painful, your sinuses clearer, and any constipation issues may resolve (due to increased fiber intake from all the fruits and vegetables you're eating). Need I go on?

People who are acutely ill, especially with abdominal issues such as irritable bowel syndrome, Crohn's disease, celiac disease, or mal-absorption syndrome, should stick to soft-cooked vegetables in the beginning and consume freshly juiced fruits (or vegetables). You need to experience some healing before taking on the added fiber of raw fruits and vegetables, and definitely stay away from nuts until your digestion improves. Nut milks and oils should be fine. Incidentally, coconut oil is very good for healing the gut and may be useful in stopping chronic diarrhea; it seems to have a beneficial anti-inflammatory effect on the gut. Again, if you are acutely ill, don't go for coconut shreds, but use a little coconut milk in a warm beverage or soup, or cook with coconut oil, which is solid at room temperature. It is suitable for high-temperature frying.

Below is an example of how making a fairly easy change can have a big impact on bladder health. Helping Rachel fine-tune her diet made a world of difference.

CASE STUDY: *Rachel's Success Story*

You did me a great service by telling me about the anti-inflammatory diet. Now I make up my meals of 80 percent alkaline and anti-inflammatory foods, and 20 percent "other" foods like proteins or starches. It has changed everything for me. I'm easily able to bring my urine pH up to normal, and I feel hugely better. I feel like I've found the missing piece. Merely avoiding the IC list of foods really didn't get to the heart of the problem for me.

There are many web and print sources where you can learn more about following an anti-inflammatory diet. Two good books on the topic are *The Anti-Inflammation Diet and Recipe Book: Protect Yourself and Your Family from Heart Disease, Arthritis, Diabetes, Allergies — and More,* by Jessica Black, ND, and *Stopping Inflammation: Relieving the Cause of Degenerative Diseases,* by Nancy Appleton, PhD.[2] (See Resources for other helpful diet books.)

What You Can Do Now

It is important to know that although the anti-inflammatory diet is a good diet to follow for the rest of your life, you may want to draw specific elements from other special diets when tailoring your nutrition to meet your individual needs. See Chapter 13 for additional diet resources. Some of the diets discussed there address health problems covered later in the book, such as vulvodynia.

After reading the last few chapters, I hope you will agree with me that carefully eliminating both common bladder irritants and foods that you are sensitive to is extremely important. I hope you also agree that eventually following a diet specific to your body's needs is key to recovering your bladder health. Throughout this process, think about the following: Are you figuring out what seems to irritate your bladder, and what doesn't? Are you following the diet that works for you individually? What are your temptations? How do you feel when you cheat? All this emphasizes the importance of tracking how you feel physically and emotionally. Consider recording your observations in a journal, or expanding your "Daily Bladder Diary" (see page 95 for an example) to include this information.

7

Stress and Chronic Pelvic Pain: Understanding Cause and Effect

This chapter discusses the role of stress in chronic pelvic pain. Both women and men can develop pelvic floor tension and other symptoms that are triggered or exacerbated by stress. We touched on relaxation in Chapter 4. In this chapter, you'll learn how to use and expand on those principles to treat pelvic floor tension, an important source of chronic pelvic pain (CPP).

The Role of Stress

The role that stress plays in all chronic disease isn't to be underestimated. Gail Sandler, an IC activist, has written that stress can be one of the major causes of a flare-up and that even *thinking* of stressful circumstances may increase bladder symptoms.[1] She considers stress reduction part of preventive medicine and tries to incorporate it into her life.

Having a feeling of control over one's life, as well as the support and understanding of family members and loved ones, is crucial to those with IC. I know this element was very important in my own recovery. Feeling loved and supported naturally reduces stress, as do a healthy diet, adequate sleep, and regular exercise. Learning to reduce the stress in your life is one of the most important factors in your recovery.

The adrenal system can be damaged by chronic stress, resulting from years of chronic pain and interrupted sleep that prevent the body from restoring and repairing this damage. I believe that future research will heighten understanding of the role that adrenal health plays in chronic diseases like IC, chronic fatigue syndrome, and fibromyalgia. Stress has already been implicated in chronic fatigue syndrome and fibromyalgia, and it is strongly associated with increasing urgency, frequency, and pain in IC.[2] The nervous system of patients with chronic pain disorders such as these (and IC) is thought to be in a state of hyperstress or hyperexcitability.[3]

Studies in both Israel and the United States have shown a strong correlation between post-traumatic stress disorder (PTSD) and fibromyalgia, with between 56 and 57 percent of those with fibromyalgia reporting significant PTSD symptoms.[4] Another recently published study examined urinary cortisol levels in women with fibromyalgia. The study compared urinary cortisol levels, as a measure of adrenal dysfunction, in forty-seven women who had fibromyalgia and fifty-eight comparable women who did not. Not surprisingly, women with fibromyalgia had significantly lower urinary cortisol levels.[5] Actually, research has shown that many people suffer from *both* fibromyalgia and IC, so, is low cortisol also found in those with IC? So far, the studies examining this issue have found this to be the case.

Dr. Jacob Teitelbaum, author of *Pain Free 1-2-3*, a popular book on treating chronic pain, has written, "[L]ower morning cortisol levels have also been associated with increased symptoms of IC." Many fibromyalgia patients see marked improvement in their IC symptoms as part of the overall treatment of their fibromyalgia. One of the treatments Dr. Teitelbaum often uses is cortisol in very low doses.[6] As we will discuss in depth in Chapter 9, chronic stress can lead to adrenal fatigue and low cortisol levels, and low cortisol is associated with inflammation, one of the primary components of IC. As we keep "pulling the threads," you'll see how many factors work together to keep us in a cycle of chronic pain and inflammation, and how we can work to reverse this process.

Research **PTSD, Adrenal Health, and Chronic Pain**

A recent study found that between 18 and 33 percent of patients with IC/painful bladder syndrome (PBS) have a history of sexual abuse.[7] The subgroup of IC patients who had this history experienced greater suprapubic (above the pubic bone) tenderness and more frequent muscle spasms of the pelvic floor than those without this history. A disturbing fact is that only *one* out of twenty-five of the women involved in this study had previously revealed her history of sexual abuse to her physician, as documented by their medical records. This is a wake-up call for clinicians: When assessing a new client with bladder symptoms of urinary frequency, urgency, and pain, or pelvic floor muscle spasms, it is important to ask whether they have suffered sexual abuse or are still suffering from PTSD, and, if so, to suggest counseling. As mentioned, a history of abuse or other psychosocial factors, perhaps resulting in PTSD, may also be associated with chronic fatigue syndrome, fibromyalgia, irritable bowel syndrome (IBS), and chronic pelvic pain (CPP)—sometimes referred to as "central sensitivity syndromes."[8]

One overlooked cause of PTSD is something called "iatrogenic abuse," or abusive actions performed during the process of carrying out medical care. Many of us, unfortunately, have experienced incidents that might qualify as iatrogenic abuse, and many victims are children. Often this form of abuse, while unintentional, can be ongoing and detrimental. In particular, when a painful procedure is performed on a child's genital or rectal area, sometimes against their will, it may be perceived by the child in the same way as rape or molestation, triggering PTSD and urological or pelvic pain disorders in later years.[9] An interesting discussion and case history is presented in the book *Stolen Tomorrows: Understanding and Treating Women's Childhood Sexual Abuse*, by Steven and Abby Levenkron. Cases of repeated urethral-dilation procedures without anesthesia or adequate pain relief, repeated probing, diagnostic procedures, and even the feeling of "being exposed" may create physiological and psychological trauma that takes years, or decades, to repair. A qualified therapist can help you explore your past medical history to see if PTSD may be a factor. I hope and pray that every medical institution

(cont'd.)

has grown more humane in the treatment of all patients, and particularly children, and I do believe they have made progress in this regard. "Patient's rights" are closely respected in most health-care settings today. Another positive factor is that parents are now less intimidated by medical professionals and are more willing to speak up on their child's behalf than were the parents of a generation ago, when it was less acceptable to "rock the boat."

Recognizing Pelvic Floor Muscle Tension

Tension in the pelvic floor muscles can compress the bladder, intensifying the feeling of pressure, urgency, and pain. Why do we tense these muscles in the first place? Here are some possible reasons:

- **We each tend to carry tension somewhere in our bodies.** For many, it is in the upper chest, upper back, shoulders, and neck, which can lead to tension headaches at the end of a stressful day. Some people clench their teeth and jaws, and, some people carry tension in the pelvic area, which causes the pelvic floor and rectal muscles to contract.

- **Many, many people with IC and other painful bladder conditions tense the pelvic floor muscles in response to pain.** It is a very common and natural response to painful stimuli to contract the surrounding muscles in an effort to contain the pain. The problem is that it doesn't work. Tensing the muscles actually exacerbates pain, especially when muscle tension becomes chronic and dysfunctional. We need to learn to stay relaxed and to breathe through the pain. Tensing our pelvic floor muscles in response to pelvic pain also tightens and shortens these muscles, which further worsens the cycle of pain and muscle dysfunction. Amy Stein, MPT, has written informatively on this reaction to pelvic pain: "The key to healing, therefore, is to let go of the tension so we can stretch and elongate the pelvic floor muscles, then strengthen the muscles around them."[10]

- **People with incontinence tense the pelvic floor muscles in an effort to hold in their urine.** This practice becomes more common after childbirth and in response to stress incontinence later in life, and it can become chronic.

- **Birth trauma or pregnancy may also trigger pelvic floor dysfunction.** Beyond any specific birth-associated trauma, pregnancy often rearranges pelvic anatomy, according to an ob-gyn I spoke with. We are truly not quite the same after pregnancy. However, physical rehabilitation can play an important role in our postpartum recovery, and it can have important implications down the road in terms of avoiding stress incontinence and pelvic prolapse as we age. In fact, in France, physical therapy is routinely offered to postpartum women who have had vaginal births, a wonderful strategy for preventing problems in later years.[11]

- **Constipation, especially chronic constipation, can weigh heavily on the pelvic floor muscles.** These same muscles, already tense, are further strained by the difficulty of passing hard stool. When we hold in stool, we are tensing the very muscles that we need to keep relaxed to resolve pelvic floor dysfunction (PFD; for more on PFD see page 136). This can be a problem especially for teachers, hospital nurses, those who work outdoors, and others who have a high degree of job responsibility yet little freedom to schedule adequate bathroom breaks. Try to go when you first feel the urge (that goes for urinating, too). If necessary, get a note from your physician that allows you to have access to a bathroom when needed. Staying regular is vitally important for anyone with PFD, and many women with IC believe it helps their comfort level, as well. The last section of this chapter includes some tips for remaining regular.

Getting to Know Your Pelvic Muscles

There are many reasons to become familiar with the pelvic muscles and their role in supporting bladder and bowel function, as well as sexual activity. These hard-working muscles also support the core of our body, maintain upright posture, and facilitate movement. However, when they become overtaxed, they can develop painful "tender points" and "trigger points" that refer pain to the bladder and other pelvic organs. Referred pain occurs when muscle trigger points transmit pain to a more distant site (see "Tender Points,

Trigger Points, and the Role of Neurogenic Inflammation" on the next page).[12] It is the very interconnectedness of these muscles, combined with their tendency to refer pain to organs such as the bladder, that requires great sensitivity and expertise in diagnosing and treating pelvic pain and PFD.[13]

Below is a brief description of most of the major pelvic muscles:

- **gluteus maximus:** We're all familiar with this one, but do you know it is the largest muscle in the human body? Besides being the "butt" of jokes, the gluteus maximus is also one of the strongest muscles in the body, as it is responsible for supporting our upright posture, controlling leg movement, and allowing for position changes.

- **levator ani:** This group of broad, flat muscles forms a sling that supports the contents of the pelvic cavity. They attach on either side of the interior of the pelvis. Dysfunction in these muscles has a large impact on bowel-related problems and may be involved in the development of pudendal neuralgia, or entrapment of the pudendal nerve, a specific pain disorder.

- **piriformis:** This is a long, pear-shaped muscle that runs at a diagonal lengthwise down the buttocks, connecting the sacrum, hip, and upper thigh. The piriformis helps with hip rotation and pelvic support, and it is frequently one of the muscles pelvic floor therapists work with to help resolve PFD. This is especially true when radiating buttock pain or tenderness also exists, which may indicate a condition known as "piriformis syndrome."

- **pubococcygeus:** Connected to the tailbone, this muscle helps to support the pelvic floor, helps to control the flow of urine, and is essentially involved in the process of vaginal birth. This important muscle is also involved in sexual arousal and orgasm in both women and men.

- **psoas:** This muscle runs lengthwise up the body, from the pubic bone and hips, through the lumbar region, to the bottom of the ribs. The psoas helps in position changes, lifting, and turning the torso.

- **sphincter ani (anal sphincter):** As you might have guessed, this is the powerful muscle that surrounds the anus and is essential for preventing bowel incontinence.

Now that you've learned some landmarks, it will be easier to understand how some of these particular muscles are involved in pelvic pain and in the development of localized pain points.

Tender Points, Trigger Points, and the Role of Neurogenic Inflammation

Tender points are small nodules found in bands of muscle that, when stimulated, are overly sensitive; they are often found in people with fibromyalgia and myofascial syndromes. Fibromyalgia patients can have these tender points scattered throughout their bodies, resulting in widespread chronic pain, often severe. Similarly, the pelvic floor muscles can be filled with tender points, making simple activities like riding a bike, having sex, or even sitting in a desk chair very uncomfortable.

Trigger points are similar, but they produce a shocking, electrical type of pain that can radiate to areas distant from the point being stimulated. In other words, trigger points can refer, or transmit, pain elsewhere in the body along nerve pathways. It is possible for an individual to have many trigger points that refer pain to the bladder. They can be found in the abdomen, at the top of the pubic bone, in the upper thigh and groin, in the vaginal wall, and in the psoas, piriformis, and other muscles in the buttocks region.

A specially trained massage therapist or physical therapist can perform specific techniques to treat trigger points in these important but sometimes overlooked muscles. You can also learn to do this yourself. A good resource is the book *The Trigger Point Therapy Workbook: Your Self-Treatment Guide for Pain Relief* (2nd edition), by Clair and Amber Davies.

How do trigger points develop, and how do they refer pain to distant sites? Some experts believe it is because of a phenomenon known as neurogenic inflammation. Neurogenic inflammation is a specific type of inflammation generated by the nervous system.[14] Many inflammatory diseases and chronic pain syndromes are thought to be driven primarily by neurogenic inflammation, including such disorders as asthma, dermatitis, migraine headache, and fibromyalgia.[15] And, recently, neurogenic inflammation has been linked to acute and chronic inflammatory conditions in the urinary tract.[16]

The neurogenic inflammatory pathway differs from inflammation caused by allergic reactions and environmental and chemical sensitivity. It is important to know that the effects of neurogenic inflammation are not necessarily limited to the location of the trigger point. The chemicals that mediate and regulate inflammation can affect distant sites and cause systemic symptoms.[17]

Afferent, or sensory, nerves are responsible for carrying a pain signal from the point of inflammation or injury to the spinal cord. Several studies have shown that capsaicin, the active ingredient in many topical arthritis remedies and in Tiger Balm and the Tiger Balm Patch, has the ability to help block the action of substance P, which is an important inflammatory neurotransmitter.[18] Through a separate mechanism, capsaicin also has the ability to desensitize sensory nerves in the bladder, thereby alleviating bladder symptoms, including pain and inflammation.

An effective program for those who suffer from neurogenic inflammation may be the following:

1. Avoid activities that produce or activate trigger points (see the next section).

2. Participate in specific therapies to alleviate trigger points.

3. Make use of topical medications containing capsaicin.

Certain substances can play a role in regulating neurogenic inflammation. We've already learned that substance P promotes inflammation, and that it can be blocked by capsaicin. Our bodies also produce an enzyme called neutral endopeptidase (NEP) that assists in keeping neurogenic inflammation in check by helping to break down substance P.[19] Harmful conditions such as cigarette-smoke inhalation and viral infections inhibit this helpful enzyme, which then leads to increased inflammation. We may experience this inflammation as rhinitis (a runny nose) or asthma. In contrast, the adrenal hormone cortisol increases this helpful enzyme, which is one way cortisol helps to control inflammation. This is yet another example of how important it is to maintain a healthy adrenal system in order to generate sufficient cortisol, which is produced in and released by the adrenal glands.

Although neurogenic inflammation may be a complicated topic to understand, it does, in fact, have practical implications that may affect your lifestyle. Some of these activities are covered in the next section.

Research   Neurogenic Inflammation

According to Dr. William Meggs, "Neurogenic inflammation is a well-defined process by which inflammation is triggered by the nervous system." Mediators such as substance P, neurokinin A, and calcitonin gene-related peptide (CGRP) are released from the sensory nerves and interact with substance P receptors on blood vessel walls to produce vasodilation (warmth and redness), edema (swelling), and, directly or indirectly, nervous system irritation.[20] Studies of cats with FIC (feline interstitial cystitis) have led to the hypothesis that this process may trigger the development of the glomerulations (submucosal hemorrhages) observed in the bladders of humans with IC.[21] (Repeated localized inflammation can lead to tissue destruction, which can in turn result in tiny pinpoint areas of bleeding in the bladder lining commonly called glomerulations, which are characteristic of IC.) A further finding from cat studies is that receptors for substance P are also found in smooth muscles and, when activated, stimulate muscle contractions. These muscle contractions may be responsible for the muscle spasms common in the pelvic floor and bladder of those with IC.

Activities That Can Activate Trigger Points and Refer Pain to the Bladder

Let's take a look at how some everyday activities can worsen pelvic and bladder pain.

Sitting

At both work and home, many of us spend the vast majority of our time sitting. Most people aren't aware that sitting can activate trigger points in the muscles surrounding the perineum and vaginal opening, and at the base of the buttocks, referring pain to the bladder. There are many very tiny, delicate muscles that can be damaged and compressed when we sit forward on our "sitz" bones, which we often do when leaning over a keyboard, riding a horse, riding a bike, and during other similar activities. It is important to change positions often and to provide adequate pressure relief in the form of cushions or pillows. You can also try a kneel-on chair or a large exercise ball for alternative sitting positions. Sometimes, it helps to turn the feet outward and separate the knees. If you want to appear more ladylike, wear a long skirt, and cross your ankles (but keep your knees apart). Get up and walk around as often as possible to stimulate blood flow to the pelvic floor. If your job requires long periods of sitting, you will need to work with your employer and with your physical therapist to come up with adaptations, including modifications of both work routines and your work environment that will help alleviate your symptoms. This is also true of men: Taking the pressure of the body's weight off the prostate at least hourly is important for men with desk jobs. Remember, you will be more productive if you are not in constant pain or running to the bathroom frequently. Your health comes first!

Biking

Bike riding, especially long distances, has significant risks for those with chronic pelvic pain, urological disorders, sexual dysfunction, and pelvic floor dysfunction. Pad your seat (or use a gel cushion), take breaks often, stretch, and stand up on the pedals as often as you can to relieve pressure. You can read more about this topic on chronic pelvic pain websites for men.

Horseback Riding

Some women have experienced bladder pain in association with riding horses. It often isn't clear whether the activity caused the pain, or whether the pain was already present and became worse with riding. Some women have needed to take a break from this activity for a while until their symptoms were brought under control.

Sexual Activity

If you're a woman experiencing a flare from PFD or IC, or have unresolved pelvic floor trigger points, having intercourse can trigger bladder pain. The discomfort may be felt during or after sex. Sometimes a female-on-top position is more comfortable and gives the woman more control over the level of penetration. However, one of the best positions is a side-lying "spooning" position with your guy behind you. In this position, all the pleasurable parts are in reach, but no pressure is placed on the bladder. There are many other options as well; it is possible to find other ways to connect besides intercourse. And don't forget nonsexual forms of affection. I don't believe in suffering for your partner, and would you really want to be with a partner who would ask you to? Frustration is a normal part of human existence, and we all learn to deal with it. Having mutual respect and allowing our partners the time and space they need to heal or deal with medical issues is essential to any healthy relationship. Your pelvic floor physical therapist or your gynecologist is probably the best person with whom to discuss issues of discomfort during sexual activity.

If the pain you feel is extreme, and the tissues that make up your vaginal opening are hypersensitive, you may have a condition known as vestibulitis, or vulvodynia. See Chapter 8, "Help with Hormones for Alleviating Discomfort," for a vulvodynia success story.

In contrast, some women find that gentle intercourse helps to relax their pelvic floor muscles, and these women benefit from regular sexual activity.

Lubricants can help many women feel more comfortable during sex, especially as we near perimenopause, which for some women begins as early as age thirty-five or forty. Lubricants can be irritating, though, if they contain propylene glycol or alcohol. One of the best lubricants is a little T and A: time and attention. I know—those two commodities can be somewhat difficult to come by in a house filled with kids, pets, homework, and conference calls, but it is important to make this effort for your partner.

Pelvic pain in men can originate from a number of causes, some of which are discussed throughout this book. According to Amy

Stein, MPT, "Pelvic pain in men is also typically associated with sexual dysfunction."[22] This is useful information to have when discussing treatment options, including medications, with your doctor. The problem may not be "in your head" or related to age or hormones, but rather may stem from a musculoskeletal problem within the pelvis, one that can be successfully treated with the help of a physical therapist. Sometimes a chiropractor is also helpful in this regard.

Kegel Exercises

Even though Kegel exercises are designed to strengthen the pelvic floor muscles, they are not recommended for women with PFD, at least in the beginning of therapy. That's because the muscles of the pelvic floor are overworked and overstressed in people with PFD. A physical therapist once told me, "An overworked, overstressed muscle is a weak muscle." You need to regain normal relaxation and blood flow to these muscles before asking them to do more work in the form of strengthening. Many physical therapists have written on the subject of pelvic floor dysfunction, and on the importance of learning to relax, lengthen, and strengthen the muscles of the pelvic floor. It is important to follow a program that helps you to learn these functions in the correct order. Relax first; *then* strengthen.

Kegels *are* recommended for women who have problems with incontinence due to weakened muscles related to age or childbirth. A physical therapist can assess your muscle strength and help you develop a strengthening program comprised of exercises specifically tailored to your body.

Pelvic Floor Dysfunction (PFD)

Over time, pelvic floor tension often becomes chronic, resulting in pelvic floor dysfunction (PFD). As discussed, pelvic floor muscles work together to support the pelvic organs, including the vagina, bladder, uterus, and rectum. When issues such as chronic pain, chronic constipation, a dropped bladder, enlarged uterus, or extreme stress are constant, chronic tension develops in these muscles, and they become shortened, tight, hyperresponsive, and prone to spasm. Although it may feel like a bladder spasm, pelvic floor muscle spasms are often responsible for many of the sudden urges to void that IC patients experience. PFD is believed to affect at least 70 percent of those with IC.[23]

A related disorder in men is pelvic myoneuropathy, a form of pelvic pain syndrome (PPS or CPPS). Caused by spasticity of the pelvic floor muscles, this condition can be effectively treated with specific physical therapy and relaxation techniques. The majority of these patients suffer from neurogenic inflammation triggered by muscle spasm (see the sidebar "Research: Neurogenic Inflammation" on page 133 for a complete explanation). For more information, check out the numerous websites on this topic that are listed in Resources.

In addition to triggering urinary urgency and frequency, PFD can manifest as heaviness or aching in the pelvis, sometimes radiating to the upper thighs or buttocks. It is similar to the feeling of a tired, overworked muscle (which in reality it is).

One of the biggest questions surrounding PFD and IC is which comes first? Does PFD cause IC? Does IC cause PFD? Or do both PFD and IC develop in response to some other cause or stressor? Dr. Robert Moldwin, an IC authority, has written, "Often some of the most pronounced symptoms of IC derive from abnormal muscle activity (in the pelvic muscle region), rather than the bladder."[24]

Many physicians I have spoken with would agree. Having suffered with IC on and off since 1995, I'm of the opinion that PFD is triggered or worsened by IC symptoms, specifically pain. That being said, once PFD exists, it is very persistent and can be continually aggravated by other factors, such as constipation (a big problem for those with PFD), sexual activity, and some physical exercises such as bicycling and swimming, particularly doing the frog kick.

Women may experience PFD differently than men do. The symptoms of PFD for both women and men are listed in Table 7.1 on the next page. There is a great deal of overlap between symptoms of PFD and symptoms of IC. As with IC, PFD symptoms can be intermittent or constant, and they may "flare" periodically, particularly after too much sitting or overdoing a particular exercise. In my experience, if you suffer from both disorders, PFD symptoms will nearly always flare up in response to an increase in IC pain. Healing bladder

TABLE 7.1: Comparison of PFD Symptoms in Women and Men

PFD SYMPTOMS IN WOMEN	PFD SYMPTOMS IN MEN
Urinary frequency, urgency, hesitancy	Urinary frequency, urgency
Pelvic and vaginal pain	Pain in the penis and testicles
Pain in the perineum (behind the vagina)	Pain in the perineum (behind the scrotum)
Pain with intercourse	Pain with ejaculation
Decreased urine flow	Decreased urine stream and hesitancy
Tight or twitchy pelvic floor muscles	Tight or twitchy pelvic floor muscles
Discomfort when sitting	Discomfort when sitting
Pain at the top of or above the pubic bone	Chronic nonspecific pelvic pain

pain and (importantly) healing chronic inflammation can reduce PFD symptoms, and certain physical therapy techniques can accelerate the process of recovering normal pelvic floor function. In addition, Eastern relaxation exercises including yoga, tai chi, and qigong, which incorporate an element of breathing, may help to moderate pelvic floor tension in some people.

One of the most annoying symptoms of PFD is urinary hesitancy, in which you experience an urge to void and then nothing happens, or there is a significant gap between an attempted void and the actual passage of urine. Learning relaxation and distraction techniques, and finding positions that relieve pelvic floor tension and spasms can help with urinary hesitancy. For nighttime voiding, keeping one's eyes open seems to help with hesitancy. Many people cannot void with their eyes closed — maybe as a result of a mechanism related to learning not to wet the bed as children?

There is one thing on which experts agree: *Straining or pushing to void urine is harmful to patients with PFD or IC.* Doing so leads to more spasticity in the pelvic floor muscles, increases pain, and furthers dysfunction. Straining or pushing to void during a spasm also increases pressure in the abdomen and within the bladder itself, which has the potential to push urine through the weakened bladder wall, intensifying the disease process in IC and greatly intensifying pain. Finally, stress and anxiety surrounding one's urological dysfunction worsens the problem of PFD. Table 7.1 gives an overview of PFD symptoms.

Addressing Pelvic-Related Symptoms

Let's take a look at some treatment strategies for pelvic issues — including both tools that will allow you to do-it-yourself and work with a physical therapist specializing in these conditions.

Coping with Urinary Hesitancy

Learn to be gentle with yourself. If you have PFD, accept the fact that for a while normal voiding isn't going to be easy. *Relax, relax, relax* — doing so is key to handling the symptoms of PFD and voiding dysfunction. While you're waiting to empty your bladder, read a magazine (now you have a medical excuse), sing a song, think great thoughts, or count backward from a hundred. Practice deep breathing and expanding the abdomen to gently stretch the pelvic floor (but don't force it).

For women with severe hesitancy, if nothing seems to be working and you're really desperate to void in order to relieve your bladder pain, assume a squatting position over a collection container. Doing this on the floor of a shower works well and avoids any problem with cleaning up accidental spills. While this suggestion may sound odd, there is a scientific reason behind it. Squatting helps to open up the pelvis, allowing the pelvic floor muscles to stretch naturally and gently and helping to prevent muscle spasticity, a hallmark of PFD. Remember that squatting is the natural position for giving birth, voiding, and defecating. It is the way women's bodies developed evolutionarily.

Certified nurse-midwife Carrie Levine has written that squatting is a healthy way to stretch the pelvic floor, tone the quadriceps, and develop core strength.[25] For women in many other cultures, voiding in a squatting position is still the preferred position. I enjoy camping and hiking, and I realized that I never had to deal with urinary hesitancy when outdoors, because I never had trouble "going" in this position. At the height of my illness, when I suffered from PFD and severe IC and experienced terrible hesitancy, this little trick was a lifesaver. My trusty container, which I kept in the bathroom cupboard, is long gone now, but I don't know what I would have done without it for quick relief.

Staying Regular

We've already discussed how suffering from constipation can strain pelvic floor muscles, so it is essential that you learn how to avoid constipation. The most natural way to aid bowel regularity is to include plenty of insoluble fiber in your diet. Insoluble fiber is insoluble in water. It isn't assimilated into the body, but rather passes through the digestive tract and is eliminated. It is very important in keeping the digestive and elimination systems regular by aiding the transit of toxic substances out of the body. This process, when operating optimally, helps to reduce the incidence of colon and rectal cancers.

Dietary sources of fiber include raw vegetables, minimally processed whole grains, and fresh fruits with skins. Increasing fiber intake slowly and adding probiotics will help to reduce bloating and gas, which can be a temporary effect of a high-fiber diet.

Below are additional suggestions for staying regular:

- Drink at least 1½–2 liters (eight to ten glasses) of water a day, or the equivalent in other liquids.

- Stimulate the bowel by drinking something hot before breakfast.

- Consume ample amounts of healthy fats, including olive, flaxseed, and coconut oils, avocados, and nuts to soften intestinal contents and lubricate transit through the colon and rectum.

- Avoid highly refined, binding foods, such as those made with white wheat flour or white rice flour, including macaroni, cream of wheat or rice cereal, egg noodles, white semolina pasta, candy, cakes, pastries, and cookies. Potatoes, eggs, and cheese can also be very constipating. Consider the BRAT diet (bananas, rice, applesauce, toast). It is often recommended following a bout of the flu or an intestinal virus because it is made of easy-to-digest simple carbohydrates and helps to firm up the stool. If these are foods you typically eat because they're bland and don't irritate your IC, they may be contributing to constipation. Try to choose more fresh fruits and vegetables with higher amounts of insoluble fiber.

- Get moving! Exercise is important in getting the bowels functioning. Try to develop a daily routine.

- If you take narcotics for pain relief, speak with your doctor about treating the chronic constipation these medications typically cause. Avoid taking narcotic medications if possible. Stool softeners can help, but they may not be appropriate for long-term use.

- Avoid regular use of laxatives, and choose a regular time to initiate your bowel movement. Typically, the body's natural time for elimination is just before or just after breakfast.

- Avoid taking calcium by itself. Calcium can be very constipating, and should always be balanced by magnesium, which can have a laxative effect. It is important to get to know your body and adjust these mineral supplements as needed to achieve a regular bowel habit. Typically, the recommended ratio of calcium to magnesium is two to one, but if you are constipated or suffer from chronic pain, a one-to-one ratio may be better for you, at least temporarily. Magnesium plays a role in moderating pain and in helping muscles relax—both important in managing IC. Considering its added role in helping to keep the bowels regular, you might consider adding this mineral to your IC recovery plan. You can find help in choosing a good brand of magnesium from the natural-health specialist at a health-food store, but it is important to know that many people prefer to take a form of magnesium that is chelated (bound to an amino acid), making it more absorbable. The preferred chelated forms may include magnesium citrate, magnesium aspartate, or magnesium glycinate. I also highly recommend ionic micronized forms of calcium and other minerals, available in liquid drops, especially for those people who have had a difficult time finding a supplement they can tolerate.

Physical Therapy

Consider working with a physical therapist (PT) who is trained and skilled in techniques of pelvic floor rehabilitation. Some PTs are also skilled in using techniques to release muscle trigger points that refer pain to the bladder. It may take a while to locate a specialized physical therapist in your area. Most of those specially trained in pelvic floor therapy (that I'm aware of) are women, but they work with patients of either gender.

There are several good books that address these issues and describe more precisely how physical therapy is used to treat pelvic dysfunction. For a mostly male perspective, read *A Headache in the Pelvis: A New Understanding and Treatment for Prostatitis and Chronic Pelvic Pain Syndromes*, by David Wise, PhD, and Rodney Anderson, MD.[26] For a more-general reference, read *Heal Pelvic Pain: A Proven Stretching, Strengthening, and Nutrition Program for Relieving Pain, Incontinence, IBS, and Other Symptoms Without Surgery*, by Amy Stein.[27]

More websites and organizations concerned with PFD are listed in the Resources section. Contact these sources for help in finding a qualified PT in your area who specializes in treating PFD. Also, take heart from Erica's story, which she shares below:

CASE STUDY: *Erica's Success Story*

I have never been sure if I have IC, although I have some IC symptoms. I have been through the entire spectrum of care—family physicians, urologists, urogynecologists, naturopaths, homeopaths, chiropractors, acupuncture, counseling, and massage. I have used all the methods outlined in *The IC Puzzle* (by Amrit Willis, RN).[28] I take lots of supplements, exercise, and practice good health. My quest to be symptom-free has persisted for six years. Early on, I tried physical therapy two times, but both times the therapist seemed to be focused on incontinence. I stopped going because if I did have IC it seemed that the recommendations and treatment I was receiving would not necessarily help with my particular symptoms.

A few months ago I decided to see a gastroenterologist about some hemorrhoids. The gastroenterologist told me that I possibly had a rectocele and cystocele (protrusions of the rectum and bladder, respectively, pressing against the vaginal walls). He said that these conditions were very likely causing my primary symptoms of urinary frequency and burning from the urethra to the rectal area. I joined an online group called "Happy Pelvis," which was started by a woman who successfully addressed pelvic symptoms with physical therapy and soon realized that maybe PT could be a puzzle piece for me.

My next goal was to find an excellent PT in my area, western Washington. I found Tina Allen through the Pelvic Pain Clinic in San Francisco, and I went to her for three months. She explained to me that I had perineal prolapse and rectal prolapse. Also, I had a hysterectomy scar that was fused to my bladder (a not uncommon condition, especially in women who may have had post-op wound infections or who developed a lot of scar tissue.) She released the scar and worked on my groin to bring blood flow into the prolapsed area. She advised me to do Kegel exercises, saying that without Kegels I could potentially need surgery. Tina explained that the perineal prolapse had resulted in constant tugging on my vaginal tissues, creating chronic urethral irritation and vaginal burning. This explains why my symptoms were always worse after a bowel movement.

After working with a physical therapist who specializes in pelvic work, most of my symptoms have gotten so much better. I still have the frequency urge, but I am working on this using the tools and techniques Tina has taught me. I feel that PT has been the one single thing that has helped me the most. However, I've never really had pelvic pain, only frequency and burning from the urethra to the rectum.

Hopefully, this will give you another view of the complexity of the female pelvic anatomy. Every person's case is different, and what concerns me is that the diagnosis of IC can sometimes be given as a diagnosis of omission. Many doctors are not as aware as they might be about the complexities of the pelvic floor, and they often fall back on a diagnosis of chronic IC, telling us to manage it as best we can. Since IC has no recognized cause or cure, it is an especially difficult diagnosis for people who might not even *have* this disorder. In my case, for example, the sensitive bladder was compromised and became irritated with the tugging caused by surgical scar tissue. Yes, there can be indicators that something is going on with the bladder, but in my case it was actually dysfunction in the tissues *surrounding* the bladder that caused my symptoms. I hope my story can be a resource for someone struggling with this pelvic puzzle.

Deep Abdominal Breathing and
Pelvic Floor Relaxation

Deep abdominal breathing and relaxation practice are wonderful ways to calm down an overstimulated nervous system, moderate chronic and acute pain, and gain control of bladder and pelvic floor spasms. Many ancient healing traditions share this element as part of a spiritual or healing practice. It is easy to learn, and it can take as little as ten minutes twice a day. It can improve sleep, produce a new sense of well-being, alleviate depression, and help you learn to deal with chronic pain.

Here's how to perform this exercise:

- Empty your bladder. Blow your nose to clear nasal passages.

- Find a comfortable place where you won't be interrupted. Turn off your phone, and if necessary hang a "do not disturb" sign on the door.

- Lie flat on your back, with heels about two feet apart. Place a small pillow under your knees if desired. Allow your legs and feet to naturally turn outward. Allow your arms to rest naturally at your sides, palms up. Alternatively, you can rest your hands lightly on your lower abdomen, over your pelvic area and bladder.

- Breathe in slowly through your nose to a count of four, allowing the abdomen to expand naturally. As breath fills your abdomen, allow your pelvic floor to gently expand outward toward your feet, slightly enlarging the space within your pelvis. The pelvic floor forms sort of a second diaphragm, a parallel to the diaphragm between your lungs and upper abdomen. It may help to picture your entire abdominal cavity as a watermelon-shaped balloon that expands and contracts with each breath. It may take a while to get the hang of this exercise, especially if your pelvic floor muscles are locked up tight. Working with a physical therapist can be very helpful.

- Exhale through your mouth to a count of four. You will begin to feel both "diaphragms" return to their normal convex positions. When you first start, your pelvic floor motion may have a jerky and unnatural feeling, particularly if you suffer from pelvic floor dysfunction, birth trauma, or severe pelvic pain. I compare it to an out-of-service elevator that hasn't been maintained properly for awhile. With practice, soon it will be expanding and contracting smoothly and easily, just as it should.

- If you feel yourself becoming lightheaded, you are trying too hard. Just relax and allow yourself to breathe normally for a few minutes, then resume deep breathing. As you gain skill in deep breathing and relaxation, try rating your overall pain and discomfort before and after your session. See if it helps you to feel better, or at least feel more grounded and in control.

Additionally, briefly applying heat in the form of a warmed rice pillow or using a heating pad set to low can help relax the pelvic floor muscles, which can help prevent the muscle spasms that wake you at night. Try this soothing technique before bedtime.

What You Can Do Now

In order to continue moving forward in your recovery, you will need to learn to relax—deeply and consciously. Let your breath fill your abdomen. Feel the pelvic floor gently expand, and then feel it spring back to its natural shape when you exhale. Notice how doing deep abdominal breathing for even a few moments, a few breaths, can help to alleviate bladder urgency and the anxiety associated with it. Feel how being in a relaxed state makes discomfort more tolerable and helps to make the pelvic floor less prone to spasm.

Assess yourself throughout the day to determine if you are holding tension in the pelvic floor muscles, keeping the pelvic floor elevated. Teach yourself to let go by breathing gently out through your mouth while you consciously try to relax your pelvic floor muscles.

In addition, you can experiment with using several effective herbs to assist you in learning to relax your pelvic floor and prevent uncomfortable muscle spasms. For complete information on herbs for the bladder, refer to Appendix B. Try chamomile, linden flower, or ashwagandha for mild to moderate symptoms and skullcap for more severe symptoms. *Note that skullcap causes sedation and has potential for danger with inappropriate use, so it is best taken under the care of a skilled herbalist.*

Finally, review your general health and daily routines to determine if any of the factors that can contribute to pelvic floor tension, such as chronic constipation or sitting for long periods of time, could be affecting your bladder symptoms. Continue to track this information in your journal.

8

Help with Hormones for Alleviating Discomfort

As part of our holistic approach to recovery, we're going to take a look at the important role that hormones play in the health of the urinary tract. We'll also discuss changes in the sex hormones estrogen, progesterone, and testosterone over time, and take a look at what happens to bladder and urethral tissues as we age, or when we experience surgical menopause.

The Sex Hormones and Bladder Health

Hormones are substances secreted by the body to stimulate the activity of specific cells. You may be familiar with estrogen, progesterone, and testosterone as the sex hormones, but insulin is also a hormone, produced by the pancreas, and cortisol is a special type of hormone produced by the adrenal glands. Hormones act as chemical messengers, and they play a significant role in the health and function of all of our bodily systems. Adequate levels of sex hormones keep the vaginal and urethral tissues well-lubricated and moist, and they also help to prevent tissue damage and loss of muscle tone. As we age, the protective function of the sex hormones diminishes, especially after natural or surgical menopause.

The drop in estrogen levels that accompanies menopause — either natural or surgical — can cause thinning of the mucosa lining the urethra, making it more prone to irritation and infection.[1] It can become uncomfortable to wear tight clothing, sit in a car, or ride a bike. A topical estrogen cream (such as the brand Estrace, or one specially made for you by a formulating pharmacy) placed at the urethral opening or on surrounding vaginal tissues can help alleviate this problem.[2] Many naturopaths specializing in treating menopausal women recommend a specially formulated topical cream containing estriol, a gentler form of estrogen (as opposed to the more commonly prescribed estradiol) that seems to specifically benefit dry, irritated vaginal tissue. Vaginal suppositories containing estriol may be another effective treatment worth discussing with your doctor. Discuss the benefits and risks of topical estrogen with your doctor. Flexible internal rings that slowly release estrogen to local tissues are sometimes prescribed by gynecologists. They are inserted like a diaphragm into the vagina just below the cervix. They can help many women with low estrogen and symptoms of vaginal dryness, but many women with IC or PFD cannot tolerate wearing them because the internal pressure causes discomfort. In addition, I believe more research is necessary to guarantee the safety and effectiveness of these products.

In addition to helping maintain healthy vaginal and urethral tissues, hormones help to maintain a healthy bladder lining. Because they contain estrogen receptors, the cells making up the bladder lining are sensitive to fluctuations in estrogen levels. Different levels of estrogen result in measurable changes in the characteristics of these cells, resulting in changes in the urge to void, smooth muscle tone, pain threshold, and the pressure within the bladder and urethra.[3] It is well known that ongoing low estrogen levels result in atrophy (shrinking and thinning) of the tissues in the vagina, urethra, and bladder, causing them to become more fragile and more easily damaged. Hormone deficiencies lead to decreases in tone and strength in the muscles of the urogenital region. All of these changes conspire to make women in perimenopause and menopause more prone to symptoms such as repeated bladder infections, and increase their general discomfort.

Dr. Elizabeth Vliet, in her popular book *Screaming to Be Heard: The Hormonal Connection Women Suspect and Doctors Still Ignore,* dedicates an entire chapter to the role that hormones play in uro-genital health. It is well worth taking the time to read and understand this information. Dr. Vliet finds it surprising that because IC overwhelmingly affects women, there is so little information in the scientific literature about the role of hormones in contributing to IC, or in its treatment. As she points out, "[E]strogen has so many effects on the bladder lining, nerves, blood vessels, and muscles that govern urinary function."[4] She lists the potential effects of estrogen decline as vaginal and vulvar dryness, itching, burning, and stinging pain, pain with intercourse, recurrent bladder infections and inflammation, urethritis, vaginitis, incontinence, painful urination, urinary frequency, and urinary urgency.

Dr. Vliet offers a number of facts that support her theory that estrogen decline is often overlooked as a factor in the development of IC:

- Researchers at Scripps Institute reported that the mean age of onset in 374 IC patients was forty-two.

- Forty-four percent of the patients in the Scripps study had hysterectomies prior to the onset of their IC. Women who have undergone hysterectomies often show premature ovarian decline and loss of estrogen, even if the ovaries are not removed during surgery.

- Surveys of IC patients have found a correlation between flare-ups and menstrual cycles, with most occurring just after ovulation and just before menses, when estrogen levels are decreasing rapidly.

However, estrogen is not the only sex hormone to affect the urethral and vaginal tissues. Testosterone, usually mentioned in conjunction with men, is one of a triad of sex hormones important to women, too. Estrogen, progesterone, and testosterone work together to maintain hormone balance. Topical testosterone cream applied in small amounts to the vaginal tissues several times weekly can help to strengthen and rebuild vaginal tissue and muscle tone. Testosterone is also often recommended to boost libido, which can be a problem for some women at certain stages of life.

What about progesterone? Although some women benefit from using natural progesterone cream to help alleviate menopausal symptoms, there seems to be anecdotal evidence that some women with IC are especially sensitive to progesterone and find that it worsens their symptoms. It is best to consult your physician, and then let your body be the judge. Remember that everyone is unique, and just because a friend may have done well with a particular hormone regimen, your body's needs may be quite different.

Menopause and a subsequent decline in hormone production isn't all bad news for those with chronic pelvic pain. Those with conditions like pelvic endometriosis and bladder endometriosis, which are aggravated by monthly surges in hormone production, should see a significant reduction in their symptoms. Now that's something to look forward to!

Pregnenolone Steal: One Reason Why Hormonal Imbalances May Exist

One possible reason for sex hormone deficiencies may again relate to adrenal dysfunction. If years of chronic pain, stress, interrupted sleep, and perhaps some unknown factor such as viral illness or autoimmune response results in adrenal fatigue, the body may need to "rob" its hormone precursor (pregnenolone) to make sufficient cortisol (the adrenal hormone), and this occurs particularly at the expense of the sex hormones. This process is known as pregnenolone steal. Hormone deficiencies can of course be precipitated or worsened by naturally occurring, age-related changes. But for women with the added factor of adrenal fatigue, the changes can be sudden, dramatic, and in general less well-tolerated than in those who have healthy adrenals, which are normally capable of taking over hormone production as the ovaries begin to slow down their production.

Overstimulation of the nervous system, whether from chronic pain, lack of sleep, or emotional stress, can also result in a decreased production of progesterone.[5] Progesterone is naturally calming, and progesterone deficiency and estrogen dominance are common in overstressed women.

Dr. Christiane Northrup, author of *The Wisdom of Menopause*, has said, "[I]f your adrenal hormones and DHEA (dehydroepiandrosterone — an important hormone precursor) levels are optimal, they can continue to produce the sex hormones for a long, long time," but if not, then bioidentical hormones may be a good choice for some women. In cases of suspected hormonal imbalance, Dr. Northrup recommends testing levels of FSH (follicle-stimulating hormone), TSH (thyroid-stimulating hormone), estrogen, progesterone, and testosterone.[6] I would also strongly recommend testing DHEA and cortisol.

Beyond the problem of sex hormone deficiencies, decreased cortisol production by the overtaxed adrenals may contribute to chronic pelvic pain, including vulvodynia, in other important ways. Studies have shown immunological changes in women with vulvodynia, including abnormal levels of tumor necrosis factor and other inflammatory markers.[7] Studies also have shown an increase in mast cells (which release histamine) in the vulvar tissue of women with vulvodynia. Low cortisol could be associated with a decreased ability to keep the inflammatory response in check. You'll learn much more about cortisol, the body's most powerful anti-inflammatory, in the next chapter.

Vulvodynia and Other Sources of Chronic Pelvic Pain

Inadequate hormone levels have also been implicated in some cases of vulvodynia and vestibulitis, chronic conditions in which the external female genital tissues (collectively known as the vulva) are hypersensitive to painful stimuli, or even to very light touch or pressure, making sexual intercourse nearly impossible. Even sitting for extended periods can be very difficult for women with chronic vulvar pain. Sometimes these conditions can occur along with IC. Supplementing with bioidentical hormones can help to alleviate symptoms in some women. Others choose to use topical estrogen creams. Still others seem not to experience much, if any, relief from estrogen supplementation and need to seek other treatments.

Most women don't like to discuss their sexual health because it is a very private and emotionally sensitive area. But here is an amazing statistic: An estimated 14 million American women have had vulvodynia at some point in their lives, although for many the condition remains undiagnosed.[8] Current estimates are that 2.4 million women in the United States have vulvodynia.[9] Doctors consider vulvodynia one of the top five reasons for chronic pelvic pain. And just because the pain of vulvodynia is "chronic," that doesn't mean it isn't also severe. I came upon a quote in Denise Foley's informative article on chronic pelvic pain that perfectly captures the way these painful disorders can control our lives: "[N]othing can be taken for granted: not walking, sitting, having sex, going to the bathroom, even wearing a favorite pair of tight-fitting jeans, which can press in all the wrong places."[10] Women with chronic pelvic pain (CPP) who wear loose stretchy pants and long skirts aren't necessarily hiding their bodies, but rather they are trying to be as comfortable as possible.

In studies of women who experience vulvodynia, whose main symptoms are usually itching, burning, and discomfort with intercourse, it is interesting to note that sexual arousal can and does occur, and many women are still able to achieve orgasm.[11] In addition, they express an interest in participating in other pleasurable sexual practices that don't involve penetration. Vulvodynia is definitely *not* synonymous with frigidity. In fact, vulvodynia can be frustrating because the normal sexual desire coexists with the often severe pain of sexual intercourse. (If you do have a low libido, it is more likely due to a hormonal deficiency, possibly even including adrenal fatigue, which we'll discuss in the next chapter.)

Vulvodynia is closely associated with a condition called vestibulitis. Vestibulitis, or vulvar vestibulitis, refers to an inflammatory skin condition producing redness and extreme sensitivity in the delicate tissues that make up the opening of the vagina. Women with vestibulitis find even light touch to be excruciating. In fact, the diagnosis of this disorder is made with the "cotton ball test" or "Q-tip test," in which a doctor lightly strokes the vulva (the soft folds enclosing the vaginal opening) with the end of a Q-tip or a cotton ball.

Many studies have looked at a sexually transmitted infection as a proposed cause of vulvodynia, but despite an extensive investigation of peer-reviewed research, there still appears to be no consensus on this. Even so, the American Congress of Obstetricians and Gynecologists stated in a 2007 patient information article that "no one knows what causes vulvodynia" and that it is "not an STD" and "not caused by HPV" (human papillomavirus).[12] Finding an accurate diagnosis might be challenging. Your best bet is to try to find a gynecological dermatologist, or at least a good dermatologist who is familiar with women's health problems.

Although the causes of vulvodynia and vestibulitis are unknown and frequently disputed, many women have reported developing symptoms following topical treatment for a yeast infection. Does the yeast infection make the nerve endings in the vulva more sensitive, or is it a sensitivity to the antifungal topical medications often prescribed? (I have not seen any reports of women who developed vulvodynia or vestibulitis after taking oral antifungals such as nystatin or Diflucan.) As mentioned, vulvodynia isn't known to be associated with sexually transmitted infections (STIs), but repeated candida infection *is* something that needs to be ruled out.[13] (While vulvodynia symptoms often include itching and burning, they don't usually involve a vaginal discharge, while candida often does.) Yeast infections with *Candida albicans* will be discussed in Chapter 10, "The Embattled Body: Dealing with Infectious Microorganisms."

It is also possible that this disorder is related to an imbalance in the vaginal flora, which under normal conditions helps to protect tissues from infection by more harmful organisms. This bacterial flora also seems to be important in maintaining a protective, lubricating, and moisturizing coating on the walls of the vaginal opening. It is interesting to note that many women with vulvodynia tend to suffer repeated yeast infections and undergo repeated topical treatments. Read Laura's story below:

CASE STUDY: *Laura's Success Story*

In December of 2005 I developed a terrible yeast infection. My doctor prescribed vaginal antifungal cream. After one application, I was on fire! Something was clearly wrong. After several attempts with creams and drugs, I switched doctors. She suspected I had vulvodynia

(cont'd.)

but wasn't sure and couldn't help me. I was exhausted and faced another month of irritation.

Simultaneously, I had been suffering from acid reflux and underwent an endoscopy. My gastroenterologist found no acid-related damage so he just put me on Nexium. At that point, I hadn't yet put the two health problems together.

I did research on vulvodynia and was scared—there was no cure, little research, and it caused suffering for so many women. I was *sure* that I had vulvodynia. I found a doctor in New York City who practiced pelvic floor rehabilitation, and I made an appointment. It took me two hours to get to his office, and he was two hours late. When I entered his office, I was scared. He asked me questions and then had me insert a device into my vagina to measure my pelvic floor strength. He thought I had low muscle endurance. I am a Pilates instructor, and I strongly disagreed with his assessment. I did as he instructed because he assured me that by following his methods of strengthening the pelvic floor muscles (which made little sense in my case), I would be healed in three months. Needless to say, it didn't work.

Six more months went by. I went to see another leading "vagina specialist" in NYC, who was also two hours late. He suggested that I needed more internal rehab and that I try Valium. After three visits to the rehab center, I developed another yeast infection, and the irritation was unbearable. My sex life, my career, even my ability to be a good mom were rapidly disappearing!

One year after my original yeast infection, I mentioned my pain to my psychologist. He was surprised because I had never spoken with him about it, and then he asked me what else was going on with my body—the first person to look at me in a *holistic* way. I described my heartburn. After further investigation, I realized that my body was acidic. I did a lot of research on acidity and pH levels. I read a book by Christopher Vasey, ND, called *The Acid-Alkaline Diet for Optimum Health*.[14] In it, he mentions "weak" acids, and he writes that some people have trouble neutralizing them. These acids can be deposited, or stored, in bodily tissues, creating pain and discomfort. I saw this theory as a possibility for treating my vulvodynia. I began to create my own low-acid, alkaline diet based on his principles. It took almost a year to become 99 percent free of pain, but it worked!

Two years after my first yeast infection, my diet got sloppy and I developed another yeast infection. This experience helped me to realize that, in my case, candida was a major culprit. Now my body's immune system is stronger, and I also understand how to attack the candida with pharmaceuticals and herbs without delay. I no longer have any vulvodynia pain, and my acid reflux, migraines, and high blood pressure are gone! It *is* possible to heal, as I did, and I want others to know that.

Treatment Options

Although pain medications are often prescribed to treat symptoms of vulvodynia, this approach does not lead to a permanent resolution. Many women look to complementary approaches and treatments, ranging from rebuilding healthy vaginal flora, to special exercises and pelvic floor therapy, to specific diets. One of the self-treatments that has provided relief for many women is a diet low in oxalates, or calcium oxalate, often in conjunction with taking supplemental calcium citrate, which helps to bind up the oxalates so they can be safely excreted.[15] Others find relief from a diet low in weak acids and other irritants, as illustrated in Laura's story above. Many of the other suggestions included in this book, such as maintaining a neutral pH and practicing stress-relieving exercises, are also helpful with cases of vulvodynia. It is also important to know that about half of the patients who've had vulvodynia are able to recover, and they no longer suffer from this painful disorder. You can find out more about a dietary approach to treating vulvodynia and vestibulitis in Chapter 13.

Research **Neurontin as a Topical Vulvodynia Treatment**

A recently conducted study evaluated the drug Neurontin (gabapentin) for the treatment of women with vulvodynia. Although long used to treat chronic pain, Neurontin can have intolerable side effects. This study looked at its use in topical form, since the pain in vulvodynia tends to be very localized. Of the thirty-five women completing the study, 80 percent showed an improvement of at least 50 percent in pain scores.[16] Others reported an improvement in sexual function. The study concluded that topical Neurontin therapy appeared to be well-tolerated and effective.

Focus on Comfort—The Sensible Solution

While you are attempting to determine if hormones may be a part of your pelvic pain picture, there are a few things you can begin to do that may help alleviate your discomfort. These concerns are particularly important in women who do not have adequate moisture levels and healthy, protective mucosa and vaginal flora—all common in women with IC and/or suffering from vulvodynia. For these women, something as simple as using the wrong soap, or any soap, may aggravate their discomfort. Consider the following:

- Feminine napkins, although old-fashioned, may feel better than tampons, at least temporarily. Look for unscented ones with the least chemical content—preferably 100 percent cotton or cloth pads.

- Stick with loose, breathable natural fiber clothing (cotton again). Consider wearing your underwear smooth side in, seam side out, and purchase them in a size larger than needed.

- During sexual activity, avoid spermicidal gels and lubricants that contain harsh chemicals. Use the most natural products you can find—check out the supply of interesting lubricants at a natural pharmacy or high-end natural-foods store. Diaphragms and IUDs can contribute to discomfort in some women.

- Also, avoid using chemical-laden feminine hygiene sprays and douches, as they may affect the pH of the vagina and upset the natural balance of vaginal flora (yes, we do maintain a population of beneficial microorganisms there, too). In fact, you can purchase probiotics made especially for this purpose, including products such as Fem Ecology (by Vitanica), Ultimate Flora (by Renew Life), and Pro-B (by RepHresh).

- When bathing, use warm water and mild soap, or forgo soap entirely on the fragile vaginal tissues. After bathing, avoid rubbing and gently pat the area dry.

- Oral contraceptives may aggravate chronic pelvic pain in some women, or they may actually improve your symptoms by helping to regulate the menstrual cycle and to moderate sudden hormonal surges in perimenopausal women, which otherwise may provoke symptoms. Work with your ob-gyn to determine whether hormonal or pain medications are a treatment you wish to explore.

- Avoid any exercises that directly press the sensitive vulva or pelvic floor against a firm surface, including (as mentioned previously in Chapter 7) horseback riding, cycling, and perhaps motorcycle riding.

What You Can Do Now

Could hormones be playing a significant role in your symptoms? When is the last time you had blood work done to check your hormone levels? Age is not an entirely reliable factor in determining when you might begin to experience hormonal changes. Depending on your general health and nutritional state, suffering from chronic stress, including chronic pain and other factors, can impact your production of hormones. Keep in mind that sex hormones also play a role in common diseases affecting women, including osteoporosis and cardiovascular disease, so, it is a very good idea to know your hormone baseline levels.

Consider the use of a topical estrogen cream, especially one containing estriol, in order to help with symptoms of discomfort with intercourse, vulvodynia, and vaginal dryness. Testosterone cream may also be of benefit to some women. Stress incontinence may lead to frequent dribbling, which could aggravate these conditions, so sometimes using a barrier cream, such as original Eucerin, on sensitive tissues may be helpful.

The phytoestrogens found in flaxseed as well as in some medicinal herbs (e.g., chasteberry, black cohosh, and Siberian ginseng) may also be useful. Flaxseed (and flaxseed oil) is recommended not just for restoring moisture to vaginal tissues but also for dry eyes (by my eye doctor, who has recommended it for hundreds of patients, with success). Topical treatment with Emu oil has provided soothing relief for some women with vulvodynia. Look for it in a specialty health-food store. Emu oil, produced from the fat of emu birds that were farmed for their meat, is high in essential fatty acids, especially omega-3 acids.

A full discussion of hormonal effects on chronic pelvic pain and the bladder is beyond the scope of this book. I do recommend reading further on this topic and discussing it with your medical practitioner or gynecologist. The art and science of understanding hormones is still developing and is not without controversy. Even some of the most highly respected authorities disagree on a variety of points. Additional information on hormones is listed in the Resources.

9

Fighting Adrenal Fatigue

In this chapter, you will learn how adrenal fatigue can lead to chronic inflammation in the bladder and other pelvic organs. I offer tips on how to strengthen and support your adrenals. Ensuring that your adrenals are in good shape will help keep inflammation in check and, for women, will help to make the transition to menopause much smoother.

The Adrenal Glands

In order to understand the significant connection between chronic stress, adrenal fatigue, and inflammation, it is important to learn a little about the important role the adrenal glands play in our bodies.

Each adrenal gland is about the size of a small walnut—pretty tiny to have such a powerful effect on the body. A critical part of our "fight-or-flight" response, they sit at the top of the kidneys and are protectively tucked just under the bottom of the rib cage in the mid-back. The outer layer of the adrenal gland, known as the cortex, is where the hormone cortisol is produced. Cortisol is a glucocorticoid hormone involved in a large number of biological processes within the body, and it does the following:

- helps (along with the pancreas) to regulate blood sugar
- supports the metabolism of carbohydrates, fats, and proteins
- moderates the body's inflammatory response

- aids in the repair of mucous membranes
- helps to control heart and blood vessel tone and central nervous system stimulation during the stress response

As you can see, because cortisol is involved in a number of important processes that directly or indirectly influence the development of inflammatory disorders like IC, maintaining a healthy cortisol level is *critical* to recovering from a chronic pelvic pain disorder.

The inner region of the adrenal gland, the medulla, is where the hormone precursor pregnenolone and the hormones DHEA, estrogen (in its various forms), progesterone, and testosterone (and other androgens) are produced. In addition to their role as sex hormones, many of these hormones have an important antiaging function. The hormone adrenaline, also known as epinephrine, is produced in the heart of the adrenal gland, along with its counterpart norepinephrine, or noradrenaline. These important hormones drive our fight-or-flight response.

Although cortisol is produced in the adrenals, it is actually regulated by the brain through a system of endocrine glands that work closely together, the hypothalamus-pituitary-adrenal (HPA) axis. The HPA axis is essential in regulating the internal biochemical environment of the body through a process known as negative feedback. For example, when a sufficient amount of a certain hormone is released, a signal is sent to the area of the HPA axis that regulates that hormone, indicating a need to decrease its output. The adrenals are well positioned to take advantage of the excellent blood supply and rapid dissemination of nearby organs and blood vessels, so that when the appropriate hormones are released, they can act quickly.

Bridging the Gap: The Adrenal Reserve

No matter what form of stress is challenging your body, it will ultimately stimulate the HPA axis and result in an increased release of cortisol, which places a temporary strain on the adrenals. One mechanism that helps the adrenals to recover is something called the adrenal reserve. Cortisol takes on several forms: It can be freely circulating, or it can be bound to proteins in circulation. It is "bound cortisol" that makes up the adrenal reserve, because it can rapidly become freely circulating cortisol when needed. People who appear to recover quickly from stress, to "bounce back," have a healthy adrenal reserve that can bridge the gap by temporarily elevating free cortisol levels in the blood without placing as much of a strain on the adrenals, thus allowing them more time to recover.

Stress and Inflammation

The negative effects of stress on our immune systems are well documented. Stress can be a precipitating factor in occurrences of simple viral infections, in flare-ups of asthma symptoms, and in reoccurrences of herpes outbreaks.[1] It can also trigger the onset of symptoms in autoimmune diseases such as multiple sclerosis and lupus (SLE). We learned in Chapter 7 that stress can exacerbate symptoms in both IC and pelvic floor dysfunction, and that stress can be an underlying factor in some cases of chronic pelvic pain. What we'll learn now is how stress allows inflammation to persist and become uncontrolled.

Inflammation occurs in all of us on a regular basis. However, the body has its own amazingly potent anti-inflammatory agent. The level of cortisol circulating in your blood, and available from your adrenal reserve, is the critical factor in controlling runaway inflammation in your body. The adrenal glands mediate the action of histamine, substance P, and other inflammatory chemical messengers by releasing cortisol. When the adrenals become fatigued and cannot keep up with cortisol production, this allows histamine to further inflame tissues, which places a greater demand on the adrenals, leading to adrenal fatigue.

How Stress Leads to Adrenal Fatigue

Stress can be defined as anything that places an added strain on the body's ability to maintain its homeostasis, or physiological balance. Such factors can include the following:

- physical, emotional, and psychological challenges
- pain
- lack of sleep
- guilt, frustration

- marital and other relationship conflicts
- failure to progress toward recovery, feelings of helplessness

These are important sources of stress faced every day by those with chronic illness. All of these forms of stress place a very real, measurable strain on the adrenal glands.

When stress is prolonged and unrelenting, as it is in anyone who is suffering from chronic illness, chronic pain, or abuse, continued high levels of cortisol are required by the body to help prevent inflammation and tissue destruction, stabilize blood sugar, moderate nervous system responses, and maintain homeostasis. Under these conditions, the adrenal reserve becomes depleted. When these high levels of cortisol cannot be maintained, and there is no significant recovery period during which the adrenals can rest and replenish themselves, adrenal fatigue results.

Adrenal Fatigue and IC

It is important to know that there is a connection between adrenal fatigue and IC. Many women with IC and/or chronic fatigue or fibromyalgia have undergone hormone testing that revealed abnormally low morning cortisol.[2] We also know that of those IC patients who have low urine cortisol, the patients with the lowest levels have more severe symptoms.[3]

Cortisol is naturally produced in a "circadian rhythm" that is important in optimal daily function, with individual dips and spikes related to drops in blood sugar and to stress. (We can help to stabilize cortisol levels throughout the day by eating regularly, including small snacks, and exercising.[4] A normal cortisol curve would begin with a rise in the early morning hours (from 4:00 AM on) to a high roughly between 7:00 AM and 8:00 AM. This provides the body with a surge of energy to get us up and moving, warming our bodies, and enabling us to forage for food, whether that means gathering fruits in the rain forest or preparing breakfast in a modern kitchen. After this time period, the cortisol level begins a gradual downward trend, as shown in Figure 9.1.

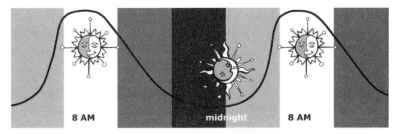

FIGURE 9.1 Cortisol fluctuation with circadian rhythm

Unfortunately, this cycle does not follow a normal pattern in those with adrenal fatigue because their bodies are unable to boost cortisol to normal levels. In essence, they are "flat-lined," skating along the bottom of the cortisol level chart. This is a graphic reflection of how it can feel to have a chronic disease, experience too many sleepless nights, and suffer tremendous pain for days or weeks at a time. Figure 9.2 shows a normal cortisol curve, which would lie between the dotted lines, and two abnormal cortisol curves, illustrating adrenal fatigue in two IC patients. This is not meant to imply that all IC patients have adrenal fatigue, but the graph clearly illustrates the finding that some IC patients have abnormally low cortisol levels in the morning, the time of day when cortisol levels normally peak, and that this is probably significant.

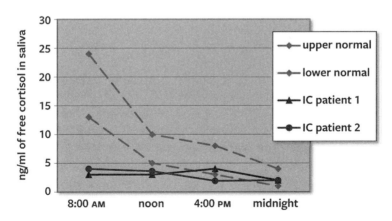

FIGURE 9.2 A normal cortisol curve and two patterns of adrenal fatigue

Why Does Inflammation Persist?

An important and perhaps overlooked question in IC and other chronic inflammatory conditions is, "What causes the inflammation to persist?" Is it the continued presence of an irritant (such as an infectious organism or an allergy)? Is it an autoimmune process, in which the body is targeting the involved tissues? Is it a failure of the body's normal controls that regulate inflammation and prevent inflammatory substances from getting out of hand? Or is it some combination of these factors? My experience from having had IC symptoms since 1995 and knowing personally the stories of many women who have benefitted from a variety of treatment approaches leads me to think that IC may, in fact, not derive entirely from a single process. Many researchers and clinicians agree. But one thing is perfectly clear: Unrelieved, prolonged stress has a detrimental effect upon the HPA axis, and perhaps upon the adrenals in particular, and this can lead to chronic inflammation.

There are several important peer-reviewed studies that support this idea. The following quote is from an article in the 2002 issue of *The Journal of Urology*:

> Little attention has focused on systemic factors that allow a state of chronic bladder inflammation to be established and maintained in interstitial cystitis cases. Abnormalities of the hypothalamic-pituitary-adrenal feedback system result in poorer regulation of the inflammatory response and are present in many chronic inflammatory and pain conditions, of which some have high co-morbidity [occur together] with interstitial cystitis.[5]

In the important study from which this quote derives, forty-eight patients with IC and thirty-five healthy, age-matched "controls" completed a questionnaire detailing their symptoms, and they deposited twenty-four-hour urine samples along with three days of saliva samples that were taken at specified intervals throughout the day.[6]

The average cortisol levels in both the urinary and saliva samples did not differ between the IC patients and the controls. However, it was noted that the IC patients who had the lowest morning cortisol levels had the worst symptoms, especially higher urinary urgency.

Those with the highest urinary cortisol reported fewer symptoms. The researchers stated that their findings imply that "regulation of the hypothalamic-pituitary-adrenal axis may be associated with interstitial cystitis symptomology." The conclusion is that the study's findings "may have treatment implications for patients with interstitial cystitis who have early morning cortisol deficiencies."[7]

Now, think over your pattern of symptoms and when they are most severe. Many women tend to have their worst frequency, urgency, and pain during the early morning hours, between 2:00 AM and 4:00 AM, which correlates with the period during which cortisol is lowest. Theoretically, after 4:00 AM, cortisol should start to rise. The usual protocol for saliva testing is to collect samples upon awakening (or at 8:00 AM), at noon, between 5:00 PM and 6:00 PM, and at midnight. I wonder what would happen if saliva samples were collected during the 2:00–4:00 AM period? My guess is that for women with severe nighttime symptoms, cortisol levels would be extremely low. With the convenience of home saliva testing, it could become a common clinical practice to test very early morning (2:00–4:00 AM) cortisol in IC patients.

The Cat Studies: A Model for IC and Adrenal Dysfunction

Cats are an excellent subject for studying IC because they can develop a similar disease called feline interstitial cystitis (FIC), or feline idiopathic cystitis. The symptoms of urinary dysfunction and increased nervous system sensitivity appear to affect cats in the same way as they affect humans. In studies conducted by Dr. Tony Buffington, a professor of Veterinary Clinical Sciences at Ohio State University, and his colleagues, autopsies revealed that many of the cats with FIC had adrenal glands that were much smaller than normal, in some cases only half the size of cats that did not have FIC.[8] Specifically, certain areas within their adrenal glands were unusually small, particularly the adrenal cortex, where the hormone cortisol is produced.

In related studies, researchers injected cats with ACTH (adrenocorticotropic hormone), the body's stress-inducing compound (similar in action to thyroid-stimulating hormone). The cats with interstitial cystitis had an abnormally low adrenal response, producing less cortisol. Thus, a *combination* of increased stress and decreased adrenal response may be significant in IC.[9]

Smaller adrenal glands in some women may be a risk factor in the development of IC. Or perhaps chronic stress in the form of severe pain, sleeplessness, and other factors related to IC result in adrenal atrophy and insufficiency. Another intriguing possibility that hasn't been thoroughly examined in relation to IC is that there may be auto-immune antibodies working against the adrenal glands themselves (see "Adrenal Dysfunction and Gluten Sensitivity," on page 169).

Dr. Richard Bercik of Yale University agrees that the connection between stress and interstitial cystitis deserves more attention, and he believes that the cat studies will lead to future examination of the role of adrenal insufficiency in human patients who have IC.[10]

Finally, Dr. Buffington has written, "Further investigation of the stress response system of patients with IC seems merited, which may provide novel approaches to therapy in some patients."[11]

FIC—Applications for Human IC Patients

Dr. Dennis Chew and Dr. Buffington write that FIC in cats is "the result of complex interactions between the bladder, nervous system, and adrenal glands [...] and the environment in which the cat lives."[12] The same may be true for some people with stress-related IC.

Changes present in feline bladder tissues included damaged bladder lining, submucosal inflammation, glomerulations (submucosal hemorrhages), and an increase in mast cells in some cats. Other important findings were increases in corticotrophin-releasing factor (from the hypothalamus) and adrenocorticotropic hormone (from the pituitary), in response to continued low cortisol during periods of stress. In other words, both the hypothalamus and the pituitary responded to the stress by asking the adrenals to produce additional stress hormone (cortisol). The failure of the adrenal glands to do so demonstrates the finding of decreased adrenal reserve among the cats with IC.[13]

Cortisol also plays an important role in maintaining "tight junction integrity" between epithelial cells—meaning that a lack of cortisol increases epithelial permeability.[14] This has implications for those with leaky gut syndrome and food allergies (both prominent in many with IC), and for those with increased permeability of the bladder epithelium. In fact, some physicians refer to IC as a "leaky bladder syndrome," in which the damaged or weakened bladder epithelium allows harmful substances irritating to the nervous system to "leak through" to the excitable muscle layer that lies beneath the protective mucosa. Activation of the sensory nerves, in turn, results in a demand for more cortisol and sets the stage for worsening adrenal fatigue.

I was very struck by this connection! It seems that cortisol is so inherently involved in many of the factors associated with IC, yet, surprisingly, few physicians seem to be aware of its potential importance. Certainly, the possibility of adrenal insufficiency was never discussed with any of my traditional allopathic physicians. I feel *strongly* that adrenal function should become a first-line test in documented cases of IC and chronic pelvic inflammation, and research supports looking in this direction.

Mild primary adrenal insufficiency (linked to abnormally small adrenal glands) can also be found in some patients with chronic fatigue syndrome or fibromyalgia (which affect many patients with IC), and in others with environmental sensitivities.[15] Several studies have shown that patients with these disorders produce less cortisol and DHEA from the adrenals, whether the cause is understimulation of the adrenal glands by the hypothalamus or pituitary, adrenal exhaustion, or some other abnormality of the endocrine stress-response system. A study published in a 2003 issue of *The Journal of Urology* concludes that for patients with confirmed adrenal abnormalities (i.e., low cortisol levels), hormone replacement therapy could be a possible new treatment for IC.[16] This is an *extremely* important bit of news that many people with IC may be unfamiliar with.

Stress and the Allergenic Response— Diet *Does* Matter

Untreated or unidentified food allergies and sensitivities are actually another, less recognized form of stress. And a significant increase in allergic response or development of allergies to new triggers is an important sign of adrenal fatigue. This is because levels of the adrenal hormone cortisol, the most powerful anti-inflammatory substance in the body, can drop very low in people suffering from adrenal fatigue.[17]

Animal studies have shown that stress triggers specialized inflammatory cells, called mast cells, to release histamine, a substance that can produce localized inflammation.[18] We also know from a number of IC studies that both mast cells and the histamine they release are found in abnormally high levels in the bladders of IC patients.[19] Cortisol is meant to regulate the reaction of mast cells and to prevent uncontrolled release of histamine and other inflammatory substances, but inadequate cortisol levels prevent this from happening. In healthy individuals, cortisol also normally prevents the accumulation of excess histamine in the body's tissues.[20]

It is very important to know that by tracking down and eliminating your food sensitivities, you will be helping your adrenals recover from the constant stress they are under. To review, the adrenals play a very important role in allergies, including food allergies and sensitivities, due to their ability to modulate inflammation and histamine release.[21] As adrenal function improves, food allergies and sensitivities *should* begin to lessen, but it may take from many months to several years to recover your adrenal health and begin to be able to eat a wider variety of foods without a return of symptoms.

Ten Foods to Avoid for Adrenal Health

Beyond the lifestyle and specific actions we can take to decrease stress on the adrenals, it is important to avoid foods that have the potential to negatively impact the adrenals. Is it any wonder that we keep hearing that the following foods are bad for us? Yet many of us continue to consume them.

In addition to the detrimental effect that sugar has on the adrenal glands, consuming sugar has a negative effect on the immune system. Eating various kinds of sugars reduces the ability of specialized white blood cells to destroy harmful bacteria and compromises our immune response. A diet containing too many simple sugars can also contribute to symptoms of hypoglycemia, a condition that places an added strain on the adrenal glands.

- white sugar/all forms of cane sugar
- white flour (and for some, all foods containing gluten)
- alcohol
- caffeine (especially important to avoid for bladder health)
- foods to which you're allergic or sensitive
- chocolate
- hydrogenated fats and oils and deep-fried foods
- fast food and other convenience foods
- junk food (high calories, no nutritional value)
- foods that have an addictive quality for you[22]

If a health professional diagnoses you as having adrenal fatigue and low cortisol, you may want to refer to Appendix B, specifically the section titled "Herbs for Adrenal Health."

Adrenal Dysfunction and Gluten Sensitivity

Prior to treating my adrenal fatigue, I suddenly developed a huge number of new food allergies and sensitivities in addition to a return of some of my IC symptoms. I also began to experience profound fatigue for the first time in my life, and my libido was adversely affected. Some people are simply born with small or weak adrenal glands. However, there is another fascinating possibility, one that may be responsible for the huge number of people with IC who have experienced improvement on a gluten-free diet.

An autoimmune disorder known as "autoimmune adrenal hypofunction" or "autoimmune hypoadrenalism," while thought to be relatively uncommon, is most closely associated with celiac disease, the hereditary form of gluten intolerance.[23] In this case, the autoimmune response mistakenly targets the adrenal glands. In fact, I was quite surprised by the wealth of information on this association, based on many studies done in Italy and Ireland, both countries where celiac disease is common. While the connection between autoimmune disorders and celiac disease is generally accepted in the United States, the case for adrenal insufficiency in relation to celiac disease does not appear to have received as much attention. Exposure to gluten in sensitive individuals has long been known to negatively affect thyroid function as well.[24] Adrenal fatigue and thyroid dysfunction are often closely associated, so if you suffer from adrenal fatigue, it is a good idea to also ask your physician for a complete thyroid workup.

Figure 9.3 demonstrates the many possible connections between adrenal fatigue and systemic effects in the body. The arrows go in

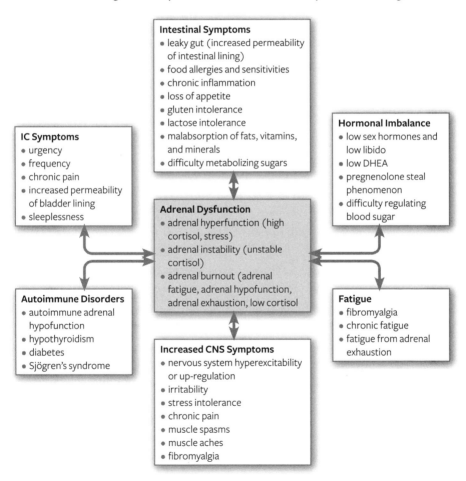

FIGURE 9.3 Possible connections in adrenal fatigue and chronic pelvic pain

both directions for a reason. Even when there appears to be a link between two imbalances in the body, it is often not clear whether there is a "causative effect" between them. Still, if you suffer from several of the problems listed below, it may be worth having a saliva adrenal function panel done. Remember that there are nonpharmaceutical interventions for adrenal fatigue, including making conscious choices to lower your stress level, to exercise, and to engage in some form of relaxation or meditation practice.

Menopause and the Adrenals

Adrenal fatigue often occurs in midlife, following the occurrence of a major stressor.[25] The normal response, after the recovery phase, would be for cortisol levels to again rise to normal, but in adrenal failure they fail to do so. What could cause an additional burden on the adrenals in mid-life? Hmm...how about menopause? In women, the sex hormones are produced in varying amounts in the ovaries, the adrenal glands, the brain, and even in body fat, but the ovaries and adrenal glands are major sources.[26] A smooth transition through menopause involves a gradual *decrease* in the production of sex hormones by the ovaries, and an *increase* in the production of sex hormones by the adrenal glands.[27]

But what could happen if there were other factors in a woman's life that prevented the adrenals from assuming this additional burden? How about chronic pain? How about chronic stress at work or living with an unsupportive partner? What about other significant causes of stress, such as divorce, financial difficulties, or the death of a parent? Coupled with the added strain that menopause places on the body, and therefore on the adrenals, a triggering event—like a severe bladder infection, an increase in food allergies, or infection with a viral or bacterial illness—could simply tax the adrenals beyond their ability to meet the increased demand.

Another factor in the relationship between adrenal function and menopause is a woman's nutritional status. Some women approach menopause after years of inadequate nutrition and emotional exhaustion.[28] Certain vitamins and minerals are essential to replenishing and nourishing the adrenal glands. Ideally, we'd obtain these essential nutritional components through our diet. In cases of adrenal fatigue, it is important to discuss with your physician what *you* can do to help your adrenals recover, both by eating an ideal diet, and by taking recommended supplements (see the section "Adrenal Recovery" on page 175 for suggestions).

A Personal Look at Adrenal Fatigue

In adrenal fatigue, as discussed, cortisol production drops and bodily inflammation becomes uncontrolled. Lack of cortisol also results in little-to-no check on the inflammatory response in autoimmune reactions, while uncontrolled inflammation leads to tissue destruction. As you can see, such a scenario could very well set the stage for chronic inflammatory disorders like IC. I had had several remissions, and I had already done much of the work of restoring and supporting my adrenals. I was in complete remission of bladder symptoms for many years — until I went through menopause.

There were undoubtedly a few other precipitating factors, one of which is that I have celiac disease. Periodically experiencing incredibly painful episodes of inflammation and tissue destruction from accidental exposure to gluten (see Chapter 5) had placed a huge strain on my adrenals. Each time my body was able to cope, but with each experience it probably took longer for my adrenals to recover. Finally, at the age of forty-eight, pushed over the edge by a hysterectomy and the loss of one ovary, I went through the final stages of menopause. Within a few months, despite supplementing with bioidentical hormones, my IC symptoms began returning. Why? Because my cortisol was very low and could not control my body's inflammatory response. In my case, the situation was revealed by testing and confirmed by the immediate positive response my body has had to treating adrenal fatigue with low-dose bioidentical cortisol replacement. However, after a little more than a year of treatment, I began to wean myself off this medication. My adrenals have recovered, and I am now able to be completely treatment-free, as long as I continue to avoid eating gluten in any form, no matter how minor the exposure might be. My IC symptoms remain in remission, as if there is no sign that I ever experienced such tremendous suffering. I'm very grateful.

Beyond IC: Other Symptoms of Adrenal Fatigue

Ten relatively common symptoms of adrenal fatigue, compiled from many public sources, are listed below:

- physical fatigue, sometimes profound
- depression and memory difficulties
- sleep disturbances
- migraine headache
- an increase in allergies or the development of new allergies
- alcohol intolerance
- low blood pressure and low body temperature
- blood sugar regulation problems (often hypoglycemia)
- low libido and hormonal imbalances
- inflammation

This closely resembles the list of symptoms I had before I recovered from IC, and I think women with chronic pelvic pain or IC would recognize many of these symptoms. However, it is *very important to avoid self-diagnosis and to be tested for adrenal fatigue before attempting to seek treatment*, especially with medicines or supplements. *You may do more harm than good if you try to self-diagnose.* The adrenals can be adversely affected by long-term use of steroid hormones, especially when taken inappropriately. Diagnosis and treatment of adrenal fatigue are discussed next.

Diagnosing Adrenal Fatigue

If you suggest to your doctor that you suffer from adrenal insufficiency, he or she may say, "That's unlikely — it's quite rare," and they'd be right — only four in one hundred thousand people have Addison's disease, the most severe form of adrenal insufficiency, and the form most recognized by traditional allopathic medicine. Addison's disease is caused by a failure of the adrenal cortex, and it can be life-threatening. In addition to problems with blood sugar regulation, sodium and fluid balance, weakness, fatigue, and nausea, Addison's often causes a dark pigmentation of the skin. However, there are many other levels of "subclinical" adrenal fatigue that may contribute to many health problems. Milder forms of adrenal insufficiency include low adrenal reserve, in which the adrenals continue to produce an adequate amount of cortisol in the absence of stress, but not enough of a reserve to cope with higher-stress periods that would ordinarily not challenge those with a healthy adrenal response. An in-depth discussion of all the levels of adrenal insufficiency is well beyond the scope of this book. However, my review of the literature has made it clear to me that stress and its relationship to chronic inflammatory disorders such as IC need a closer look.

The question of whether adrenal fatigue may be affecting *your* health is a discussion you should have with your physician. If your physician isn't interested in having this discussion, then you could consider seeing a naturopath who specializes in hormone testing and/or managing chronic illness.

Testing for adrenal insufficiency is an established and useful diagnostic tool that might have important implications for poor regulation of inflammation as well as for general health. The first step is to check for a low cortisol level, in combination with checking the levels of other hormones including DHEA, progesterone, estrogen, and testosterone. This is easily done with a safe, reliable, and cost-effective serial saliva test, with four samples taken at specified time periods throughout the day. Your physician often stocks these kits in the office, and she or he can provide one for you to use and then mail to the laboratory. The laboratory will perform the tests and send the results to your physician, who will discuss them with you. The whole process takes a week or two, and can be repeated every few months to track your recovery. It isn't expensive and may even be covered by your insurance.

In fact, you do not need a doctor to order the test, but the results will be of little value without a physician to interpret them, develop a treatment plan, and support and monitor your progress.

Blood tests, including an ACTH challenge, which stimulates the adrenal glands to produce cortisol, may be indicated later, but a serial saliva test is a good first step.

Adrenal Recovery

The power of stress to affect our health can be seen in the curious fact that people with chronic pain and disorders such as IC will often experience some relief while on vacation. This can lead to questions about possible environmental illness or other factors present in their ordinary home life. But what really may be playing the more significant role is a change in *lifestyle* rather than a change in *environment*. You absolutely must take the time you need to heal, alleviate stress, transform your lifestyle, modify your diet, and take control of your life — something that may indeed be easier to achieve while taking a break from work and the demands of daily life.

The good news is that you can recover from adrenal fatigue by using many of the actions and treatment methods discussed in the previous chapters and with the help of a skilled practitioner who specializes in treating adrenal fatigue and chronic illness.

Every part of this book is dedicated to resolving adrenal fatigue in its own way, from addressing pain, to discovering and eliminating food allergies, to promoting stress reduction through exercise and relaxation, to achieving hormonal balance. These healthful practices are the heart of any recovery plan for chronic illness, including one for IC and chronic pelvic pain.

Adrenal health affects nearly all the body's tissues and systems. Our ability to recover from IC by focusing on *any one* of these factors is one of the reasons that IC has proven to be such a complicated disorder to treat. Alleviating pain, even temporarily, and promoting restorative sleep helps tremendously to lessen the adrenal burden. Following a healthful diet, achieving relaxation on a regular basis, eliminating food allergies, and balancing hormones all have the potential to help us move closer to balance and take the load off the overtaxed adrenals.

Take a moment and just imagine how doing *all* of these things would benefit your adrenal health. Together, these actions would begin to decrease inflammation, allow your body's nervous system to wind down, and generally begin to reverse the process that leads to IC and chronic pelvic pain.

Any program of adrenal recovery must incorporate lifestyle changes: Avoiding stress and dealing with stress in healthy ways, such as exercise, relaxation, and meditation, is essential. Eating an anti-inflammatory diet, free of sugars and alcohol, is essential. Further supporting the adrenals with some of the specific herbal teas listed in Appendix B is also a very helpful and pleasant way to promote recovery from adrenal fatigue or chronic illness.

Beyond these elements, the suggestions presented below may be helpful.

Supplements for Adrenal Fatigue

Many sources recommend using specific nutritional supplements to help support and heal the adrenals, but be sure to check with your physician before beginning any supplement regimen. People with kidney dysfunction, for example, may not be able to tolerate certain minerals and may need to control their protein and sodium intake. Anyone with a suspected hormone imbalance needs to undergo appropriate testing before self-administering hormones or their precursors.

It is best to consult with a qualified health practitioner who specializes in treating adrenal fatigue; otherwise, follow manufacturer's directions, and remember to *try only one supplement at a time.*

- Maintain an optimal ratio of omega-3 and omega-6 oils. For most people, this means increasing intake of omega-3 oils from food sources, fish oil, and flaxseed oil. Follow your practitioner's guidelines.

- Vitamin A — follow the manufacturer's recommendations.

- All the B vitamins, but especially biotin, vitamin B-5 (pantothenic acid), and vitamin B-6 (pyridoxine). Those with profound fatigue may wish to inquire about intramuscular injections of B vitamins.

- Vitamin C — necessary for many bodily functions; 1,000 to 2,000 mg/day, as tolerated. Buffered or ester-C products are particularly recommended for those with bladder pain.

- Magnesium — 500 mg/day (balance with calcium).

- Zinc — 50 mg/day.

- Coenzyme Q10 — if tolerated; follow the manufacturer's suggested dosage.

- L-glutamine — an amino acid that helps to repair increased intestinal permeability (leaky gut), and L-carnitine, which has a protective effect on the nervous system, and also helps to support adrenal health. L-tyrosine may aid adrenal gland function. Dosage recommendations vary, and excess intake may cause GI upset.

- DHEA and/or pregnenolone — may help with hormonal support. Avoid exceeding recommended dosages and use the lowest effective dose of these hormones.

- Melatonin or 5-hydroxytryptophan (5-HTP) may help with sleep and allow the adrenals to rest and recover. Melatonin has also been shown to increase secretory IgA, which is the first line of defense in mucous membranes, and may be helpful, along with L-glutamine, in repairing increased intestinal permeability (leaky gut).[29] Use the manufacturer's recommended dosage.

- Herbs that nourish and support the adrenals, such as astragalus, ashwagandha, borage, and rhodiola. Licorice root and Siberian ginseng are often suggested but can be too harsh for the IC bladder, and licorice should not be taken long-term. Please refer to Appendix B for more information on herbs for the bladder and the adrenals.

Below, an IC friend shares her story of healing through adrenal recovery.

CASE STUDY: *Kimberly's Success Story*

We all want an answer as to *why* we have interstitial cystitis, and we *really* want a miracle—a healing, a cure. After twenty-six years of living with the disease, I may be one of the lucky ones who stumbled upon both. At age fifty-one, medical knowledge may have advanced enough to finally point to the cause of inflammation, aching muscles, and chronic vaginal infection I have been living with for so long.

When I was first diagnosed with IC at age twenty-five, I had already learned that chronic candida yeast infections and bacterial vaginosis were a primary cause of bladder pain and inflammation for me. If I had

(cont'd.)

a vaginal discharge of any kind, I also had horrible, unrelenting bladder pain. My bladder wall had likely been weakened by a chlamydia infection that went undiagnosed for over a year prior to the bladder pain beginning. In addition, during this time period, I developed a complete intolerance to alcohol. Forty-eight hours after drinking any kind of alcohol, my bladder pain would flare, with symptoms lasting as long as a month. My body was exhausted, and nearly every muscle ached. I was twice diagnosed with fibromyalgia, although I knew that my muscles only ached when I also had bladder pain. Waking up in the morning was terribly difficult, and I was often irritable and unable to cope with stress.

For years afterward, I learned as much as I could about IC, and I developed a routine that helped me to lead a relatively normal life. Preventive medication for yeast and bacterial vaginosis infections and a low-acid diet with no sugar or white flour had helped to keep my bladder calm and mostly free of inflammation. But, at fifty-one, menopause suddenly took a devastating toll on my bladder. The lack of estrogen that came with menopause seemed to bring my IC back to an intolerable level. In an effort to begin restoring my health, a naturopath tested my allergies and we learned that I could not tolerate dairy, soy, ginger, and basil. I started on bioidentical vaginal suppositories to heal the tissues in my urethra and vagina. As I described the muscle aches, alcohol intolerance, exhaustion, and depression, she also suggested a saliva test to determine the levels of my sex and adrenal hormones. My sex hormones—estrogen, progesterone, and testosterone—were doing fairly well, considering my menopausal status, but the level of cortisol was low enough to suggest a cause for most of my symptoms. My morning cortisol levels—which should have been between 7 and 10 ng/ml (nagstroms per milliliter)—were only 1.9 ng/ml at their highest point in a twenty-four-hour period. My adrenal glands had almost stopped functioning.

What I have been living with for twenty-five years is often called "adrenal fatigue," or, at my low levels, "adrenal exhaustion," or subclinical Addison's disease. My childhood and early adult years before IC had been filled with chronic stress and serious illness. Looking back, as my adrenal dysfunction and bladder inflammation progressed, I realized that I had worked long hours, married and divorced an alcoholic, and raised two children as a single mother. I was the *definition* of adrenal exhaustion. My poor body lacked the social and emotional support, good nutrition, and relaxation that allow the adrenal glands to rest and recover after periods of stress. Inflammation often goes unchecked when cortisol levels are low—a clear explanation for my bladder inflammation. The development of numerous food sensitivities, which I experienced, is also consistent with adrenal fatigue.

My naturopath prescribed food-based B vitamins (Nutriplex), buffered vitamin C, sublingual B-12, chromium, biotin, and the antioxidants vitamin E, selenium, CoQ10, and lipoic acid in an effort to nourish my adrenal glands and correct the hypoglycemia that often accompanies adrenal exhaustion. I worked to find supplement brands that my bladder could tolerate. She prescribed Wise Woman Herbals solid extract licorice (¼ teaspoon twice daily) to stimulate production of cortisol. I felt better immediately, with greater energy and stress tolerance, and I also experienced improved, more restful sleep. A bladder flare, however, later sent me back to her for more support. We made the decision that I would try 10 mg of a prescription medication called hydrocortisone (5 mg at first waking, 5 mg by noon). This amount of synthetic corticosteroid is considered a replacement dosage, just as a small amount of thyroid hormone is used as a replacement for inadequate thyroid hormone in cases of hypothyroidism. Eventually, with the help of my doctor, I will transition back to natural substances that help stimulate the adrenal glands to produce cortisol, and I will continue to support my adrenals with the supplements my naturopath suggested.

Within one week of my beginning the hydrocortisone, every single symptom I had vanished. I felt like I had been given a new body and a new lease on life. The inflammation is gone, the vaginal infections have yet to return, and I feel energetic, optimistic, and relaxed. Although cortisol is stimulating, I do not feel restless or irritable, because I am only replacing what my body lacked. I have allowed myself a bit of sugar here and there with no repercussion, although I plan to maintain my previous healthy diet to further support the healing taking place in my body.

I believe it is necessary to work with a naturopath who uses saliva testing in order to obtain accurate cortisol readings, as they naturally fluctuate throughout the day. Many allopathic doctors have yet to acknowledge adrenal fatigue as a treatable condition, and they generally do not use saliva testing.

What You Can Do Now

You've learned that you must monitor yourself carefully, treat and feed yourself well, and adopt a lower-stress lifestyle. You should include time to exercise, seek out supportive friends and family members, and allow yourself time to heal. Continue to track your progress in these areas as you begin to see some positive results from dietary changes, the use of helpful herbal teas, and lifestyle changes, such as reducing stress.

Remember that people with IC may have genetic or developmental differences in their ability to handle stress. Certainly within my own family, this seems to be the pattern that exists. Maybe this isn't true in your case, but certainly *any* plan for recovery from chronic illness should include all of the above elements. Here's a quote from the late noted-herbalist Michael Moore: "Virtually *every* urinary tract problem starts from metabolic imbalances, and at every stage I urge you to examine personal patterns of stress and [...] make appropriate changes in diet so the conditions underlying the problem are alleviated."[30]

Hopefully you've begun to feel a bit better, or a whole lot better, depending on your individual pathway to recovering from IC. For those who feel they've not yet found their answer, there's a lot more to cover, which we'll begin in Part III, "Further Along the Road to Recovery: Suggestions for Those Who Are Still Struggling." In this second-phase recovery plan, we'll cover such topics as Lyme disease and its associated pathogens, occult bacterial infections, candida yeast overgrowth and gut dysbiosis, other sources of chronic pelvic pain, complementary therapies, and measuring successful recovery by your own standards. Remember that other disorders may exist in addition to IC or other forms of chronic pelvic pain, and that in a holistic approach, *all* elements need to be addressed.

PART III

Further Along the Road to Recovery

Suggestions for Those Who Are Still Struggling

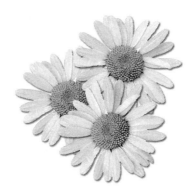

10

The Embattled Body: Dealing with Infectious Microorganisms

It is heartbreaking to be diligently doing all the tedious things you're supposed to do to get well and yet feeling as if you're not getting anywhere. I understand your frustration, because I've been there, too. If that's your situation, then Part III of this book is especially for you. Please don't give up hope. Your answer is going to be a bit more of a challenge, but you can find it, hopefully, somewhere in the pages ahead. This is why I encourage you to "leave no stone unturned" in your quest for a better bladder and improved health.

The goal of this chapter is to rule out the possibility that specific microorganisms may be contributing to your chronic health problems and preventing your recovery. We've mostly been dealing with the macroscopic level—things we can see with our eyes. However, to find your answer, you may need to look deeper—into things that can only be seen with a microscope. This first chapter of Part III will introduce some additional potential problems you may need to investigate, but for the most part I consider these to be secondary complications of a system that is overstressed and out of balance. A good analogy is: "Even after you fix the wagon wheel, you still need to move the boulders blocking the way before you proceed over the mountain."

Occult Bacterial Infections

You may be thinking to yourself, "I've had so many tests for bladder infections that they couldn't possibly have missed anything. I've even been on prophylactic antibiotics." However, could it be possible that your symptoms, at least some of them, are caused by an occult (hidden) bacterial infection? The answer is "maybe," and therefore it is definitely worth ruling out this possibility.

The Standard Urinalysis and Culture

The standard urinalysis and culture performed in your doctor's lab is a process designed for rapid, efficient detection of the most common types of bacteria found in urinary tract infections (UTIs). Results of a standard urine culture are usually available in a matter of days. Your physician, especially a good urologist, will also usually examine your urine under a microscope. The majority of all urinary tract infections are caused by *E. coli* (*Escherichia coli*), a gram-negative bacterium commonly found in the large intestines and consisting of many different strains, some of which can become pathogenic, or virulent. These virulent strains of *E. coli* can cause gastroenteritis, peritonitis, and septicemia. Certain strains produce the toxins that cause the violent gastrointestinal symptoms of food poisoning.

Even these common urinary tract infections may be serious, may progress to your kidneys, and should be treated by a medical professional. However, there is another type of infection, caused by a different type of bacteria, which is more difficult to detect with the standard approach used in virtually every lab and hospital in the United States.

The Urine Broth Culture

Before the newer, more efficient method of urinalysis and rapid culture became the accepted standard, urine was sometimes cultured in a broth, or liquid medium. This is known as a urine broth culture. It takes longer to grow, but if you think about it, growing bacteria in a broth medium more closely approximates the environmental conditions that exist in the bladder. And this is apparently the key to growing the kinds of organisms that sometimes exist as occult infections in people with IC. A urine broth culture is held at a controlled temperature for a longer period of time to allow bacteria to grow. In some laboratories, the specific species that grow are more important than the colony count (the number of microbial organisms present). This sometimes gives rise to criticism that these bacteria are contaminants, and there is some controversy regarding this approach.

Some of these organisms include *Staphylococcus aureus* and *Enterococcus*, both gram-positive bacteria, and, less commonly, *Serratia*, a gram-negative bacterium. All are detectable when grown in a broth culture. Can these organisms cause the symptoms found in people with IC? The answer is "Yes." Do these organisms actually cause IC? We don't know for sure. And we certainly don't know that a bacterial pathogen is responsible for *all* cases of IC. There simply haven't been enough studies done to confirm the infectious organism cause of IC, but many scientists also feel there haven't been enough studies done to rule out an infectious cause.

More on Occult Infections

In a study published in 1994, a researcher with the University of Maryland School of Medicine wrote, "[I]nfection has not been properly ruled out as a factor in the development of interstitial cystitis."[1] He goes on to explain that ruling out infection in IC would require special techniques to search for microorganisms in *both* bladder tissue and urine, something not commonly done. An infectious process isn't necessarily in conflict with other theories regarding the cause of interstitial cystitis, including autoimmune disease, increased bladder permeability, or even some as yet unknown genetic predisposition.

In a study done in Switzerland, women with a history of urinary urgency, frequency, and chronic pelvic pain, and those with a history of recurrent UTI, were examined, tested for infectious organisms, and treated with doxycycline and, in some cases, also with a vaginal antibiotic. The study's conclusions were significant: 71 percent of the women in the study experienced either a decrease or resolution of their symptoms.[2] It is worth noting that a diagnosis of IC was *not* necessary to participate in the study, and subjects had a wide array of symptoms. Still, this study does lend credence to the possibility of an infectious organism in the "disease process" of IC. I state it this way intentionally, because it remains unclear whether any infectious organism has a "causative" role in every case of IC.

One theory is that occult infections are opportunistic, secondary infections that arise due to an already impaired bladder mucosal lining, in combination with a weakened immune system, and that they wouldn't have been able to take hold in a normal bladder. A normal, healthy bladder mucosa has the ability to slough off bacteria before they can attach and create a localized infection. However, if something damages the bladder, creating an opening or weakened area in the bladder lining, then a bacterial infection can take hold. The bladder can be injured by a previous infection, sexual trauma, an invasive procedure such as a cystoscopy, or possibly by an inflammatory process triggered by eating gluten or another substance that provokes an allergic reaction. As you've read in earlier chapters, gluten-associated damage often causes problems in the mucosa of other parts of the body. Why not the bladder?

It is your decision, but if you're stuck and aren't getting any better no matter what you do, consider having a broth culture performed with the support and guidance of a local physician so you can at least rule out this possibility.

Practical Information on the Urine Broth Culture

You do not need a doctor's order to have the test done. However, you do need a doctor, physician's assistant, or nurse practitioner to prescribe the antibiotics with which to treat any infection the test reveals, and it helps tremendously to have the help, support, and guidance of a physician or skilled urological nurse-practitioner to help you in this process. Occult bacterial infections that are really entrenched, having existed sometimes for many years, may require long-term antibiotic use, which, in turn, will undoubtedly create temporary gut dysbiosis and a flare in naturally occurring *Candida albicans* (a common species of yeast). This will usually need to be treated by prescription antifungals such as nystatin or Diflucan (fluconazole), along with probiotics to rebuild the intestinal flora. (You'll learn more about this in the section "Candida Overgrowth," below.)

Other infectious organisms that may be associated with IC-like symptoms are mycoplasma, which is associated with pelvic inflammatory disease, and ureaplasma, which may be responsible for nonspecific urethritis, or inflammation of the urethra. These organisms may be difficult to detect unless a practitioner specifically looks for them. You can request that your physician test you for these specific organisms, and if infection is present, it can be treated with antibiotics.

You can obtain a urine broth culture by ordering it from United Medical Labs, in McLean, Virginia, or from John Toth, DO, in Concord, California. Dr. Toth treats many patients with IC using a *holistic* approach. He was also kind enough to review the final draft of *The Better Bladder Book* and to write the book's Foreword.

You can arrange with either facility to mail a report showing any species of bacteria cultured from your urine using the broth method to you or to your physician. Insurance may or may not cover the cost of the test, which is in the neighborhood of $130.00. (For contact information, see Resources.)

My Experience

I went through the experience of having a urine broth culture performed, followed by long-term antibiotic treatment. The side effects, including candida overgrowth, were not pleasant, but I would do it again if I had to. For at least five years I'd endured what felt like a burning charcoal briquette in a localized part of my pelvic area. Nothing would touch this pain, not even strong narcotics. It was always present, and when I was in a flare, I would often be tearful and gasping from the severe pain. Even at night I was not free from this pain, and I would sometimes dream that someone was stabbing a knife into my lower abdomen. After six weeks on antibiotics, this localized, severe pain was virtually gone and has never returned. Did the antibiotics cure my IC? Unfortunately, no, because I had more work to do. The frequency, urgency, and urinary hesitancy, and my general crankiness remained, and I experienced a few flares, but my pain level never again reached above a seven or eight, and usually it was below a three most of the time, which was a great deal easier to live with.

After undergoing a little more than two months of antibiotic treatment, my continuing improvement stalled. It then took a few more years to realize just how sensitive my bladder was to gluten before I was able to go into a long-term remission. Celiac disease and gluten intolerance can unfortunately cause malabsorption of the proteins needed for tissue repair, so it can take quite a long time to heal from IC, even on a strict gluten-free diet.

Testing Sexual Partners

Whether or not to test sexual partners for occult infections is something we need to seriously consider.[3] I did encourage my husband to have a urine broth culture performed, and, not coincidentally, he had the same bacterial infection that I had. (Due to unusual circumstances, he used a different lab than I did, and his test was done several months after I began a regime of long-term antibiotics.) I chose to do this for two reasons. First, he had also begun to have some bladder symptoms for the first time, which really scared both of us, and second, because after taking long-term antibiotics and then battling candida, I really did not want to be reinfected if he were a carrier of an occult infection. We both had the broth culture testing performed, followed by the antibiotic treatment, followed by a repeat broth culture test. Then, we worked to get the resulting gut dysbiosis under control, which took from six months to a year.

Bacterial Parasites and Occult Urological Infections

In 2001 researchers at Vanderbilt University announced that they had discovered a potential role of an infectious organism, *Chlamydia pneumoniae* (also called *Chlamydophila pneumoniae)*, in the disease process of IC. One of the study's principle researchers, Dr. Jenny Franke, described a "statistically significant correlation between IC and infection with *C. pneumoniae*."[4] This bacterium is a major cause of pneumonia, as its name indicates, and it has a respiratory means of transmission (i.e., the organism is spread when a person inhales droplets from an infected person's cough). It should be noted that *C. pneumoniae* is not the same organism that causes the common sexually transmitted infection chlamydia (*C. trachomatis*).[5] *C. pneumoniae* is a very common respiratory pathogen—nearly all of us have been exposed to it by the age of adulthood — and it causes about 10 percent of all pneumonia cases worldwide.[6] The initial symptoms are no different from more typical pneumonia symptoms (cough, fever, difficulty breathing). So what's the connection with IC?

Because this organism is known to cause chronic secondary infections, Vanderbilt University's Drs. Stratton, Alberts, Mitchell, and Frank decided to look for its presence in patients with IC. Their original study analyzed the urine of both IC patients and controls for the presence of *C. pneumoniae* and found that 81 percent of IC patients were positive, in contrast to only 16 percent of the controls! This strongly suggests an important correlation, and could point to a potential role of an infectious organism in the development of IC. The Vanderbilt group went on to biopsy the bladders of seventeen patients who had IC, as well as those of six controls (who did not have any symptoms of bladder irritation or recurrent UTI).[7] The biopsy results were again statistically significant, paralleling the findings in the urine tests: Eighty-two percent of IC patients had positive tissue cultures, in contrast to 16 percent of the controls. Other major research centers around the country, including Johns Hopkins and the Mayo Clinic, have begun looking at the role of *C. pneumoniae* in chronic inflammatory diseases.

C. pneumoniae is a bacterium. We have many powerful antibiotics, so what's the problem? There are several. First, *C. pneumoniae* is an obligate intracellular parasite. This means that it does not have the ability to produce its own energy; in order to survive and reproduce, it steals energy from the body's cells. In particular, the organism is especially drawn to infect the cells lining the blood vessels. The lungs are rich in blood vessels, having the critical job of exchanging oxygen and carbon dioxide from the air we breathe. In active infection, our immune response involves releasing specialized cells to surround the invaders and ultimately gobble them up and annihilate them. But *C. pneumoniae* is very hard to kill, and instead, these specialized disease-fighting cells can end up spreading the infection to more distant parts of the body, sometimes causing "occult" (also known as "cryptic," or hidden, infections).[8] These terms refer to bacterial infections that may be overlooked or are difficult to find using standard testing practices, or even those that may be difficult to detect in certain inactive forms of their life cycles.

As part of our body's immune response system, any time there is inflammation, new blood cells are formed in that area, and *C. pneumoniae* is specifically drawn to these areas. This can mean that an insect bite, a viral infection, or an ordinary urinary tract infection can become the locus of a new, persistent, cryptic infection with *C. pneumoniae*. Vanderbilt researchers hypothesize that this is the mechanism by which this pathogen is implicated, not only in IC, but also in other chronic inflammatory diseases, including rheumatoid arthritis and fibromyalgia/chronic fatigue syndrome.[9]

Unfortunately, once these secondary infections develop, *C. pneumoniae* is difficult to eradicate, necessitating long-term treatment, often with a regimen of several antibiotics taken simultaneously.[10] This organism is also difficult to detect using routine laboratory methods, and in order to make sure that the organism is totally eradicated, repeat testing may be required in every stage of its complex life cycle.[11] Another complicating factor is that the bacterium itself produces "endotoxins," which can cause symptoms such as inflammation, pain, depression, and chronically low energy, symptoms that are magnified when large amounts of the organism are killed, releasing large amounts of their endotoxins at once.

In addition to research linking *C. pneumoniae* to IC, an Italian study published in 2003 examined the presence of this occult infection in a group of forty men with a history of prostate pathologies including BPH, chronic abacterial prostatitis, and prostate cancer. The significant majority—87 percent—were positive for *C. pneumoniae* DNA. Of the ten patients who consented to prostate biopsy, 100 percent positively demonstrated the presence of *C. pneumoniae* (representing all three prostate disorders). The researchers concluded that future study of this microorganism in relation to prostate disorders is very important and suggested several avenues for further research.[12]

It is interesting to read the above study and to know that testing for *C. pneumoniae* is not yet part of standard practice in diagnosing and treating IC. It is not clear whether this is due to some perceived fault of the study, failure by others to replicate the results of the study, or some other reason.

Testing for *Chlamydia pneumoniae* is a complicated process, involving deciphering the organism's DNA and testing for specific antibodies. It would be best to try to locate a physician who is a specialist in this area. Since this organism is also implicated in fibromyalgia and chronic fatigue, a clinic specializing in these disorders is one place to start your investigation.

If you're not getting anywhere in your search for answers and your IC is still progressing, talk with your physician. It is important to understand that long-term antibiotic treatment is controversial because it involves very real risks, and it is not considered the standard of care. It is also possible to become reinfected; eradicating the existing infection is no guarantee that you will not develop another one in the future. Your physician may advise against the long-term antibiotic approach, but hopefully she or he will at least be willing to engage in a discussion with you.

There are some articles relevant to the long-term antibiotic approach to treating IC listed in the Resources. Viewing these articles and other information may help you to learn more about the treatment of occult bacterial infections and determine if this is an area worth exploring in your particular case.

Bladder Symptoms in Lyme Disease

Speaking of occult infections, here is another possibility to rule out. I have read of many people who experienced chronic bladder problems similar to IC before being diagnosed with Lyme disease. One general description of these symptoms is "irritable bladder—with trouble starting and stopping, or interstitial cystitis-like symptoms."[13] Usually, bladder problems were not the only symptoms present, but rather they occurred along with chronic fatigue, fibromyalgia or chronic muscle pain, joint pain, and neurological problems. Since I have a history of chronic headaches and bladder symptoms, and had lived in areas where Lyme disease is common, my physician suggested that I also be checked for Lyme, but my tests were negative.

Lyme disease is caused by a tiny tick-borne parasitic bacterium called a spirochete—*Borrelia burgdorferi*. The ticks that cause Lyme disease are often carried by deer, and then transferred to other animals and humans that come into contact with them. Walking through long grass is a common method of transmission.[14] This spirochete has been found both in bladder biopsies and the urine of patients with Lyme disease.[15] There is some evidence that infection with the organism that causes Lyme disease can cause symptoms that mimic IC or that Lyme infection negatively affects the immune system and predisposes its victims to IC-like symptoms. Studies done with mice showed that mice infected with *B. burgdorferi* showed significant pathologic changes in the bladder, including an increase in the number of blood vessels, thickening of the vessel walls, immune system-induced changes, and inflammation. Nearly all (93 percent) of the mice examined in the studies had spirochete-induced cystitis.[16]

Although there is ample anecdotal evidence of people who have recovered from IC-like symptoms after long-term antibiotic or complementary treatment for Lyme disease, the most definitive study to date does not make this relationship entirely clear. Tests for various types of antibodies to Lyme disease were studied in fifty patients with IC. Patients with positive antibodies were given bladder biopsies. None of the patients with positive antibodies had *active* Lyme disease, but 8 percent of patients with IC had antibodies indicative of *past* infection with Lyme disease, while only 2 percent of the control group did. The researchers concluded, "These results indicate that persistent infection of *B. burgdorferi* has no role in the etiology of IC. On the other hand a connection with a past *Borrelia* infection and IC isn't excluded."[17]

Other Symptoms of Lyme Disease

B. burgdorferi infection may cause initial flulike symptoms with fever, headache, nausea, jaw pain, light sensitivity, reddened eyes, muscle ache, and a stiff neck. A bull's-eye rash is characteristic but may go unnoticed; other rashes are common, but the tick itself is so tiny as to be hardly noticeable.

Lingering symptoms of Lyme disease are varied and can include chronic head and muscle aches, neurological symptoms, vision and hearing disturbances, gastrointestinal symptoms, and worsening allergies. Bone and joint pain as well as fibromyalgia-like symptoms are very common. Lyme disease is also linked to a condition known as Bell's palsy, a type of facial paralysis. Swollen lymph glands, unexplained fevers, and symptoms that migrate to different parts of the body over a period of time are additional symptoms physicians look for.[18]

It is a good idea to see a practitioner who has a holistic perspective and who will therefore look at all of the symptoms you are experiencing as a whole rather than in isolation. Diagnosis can be difficult. Still, in the past two decades, physicians have become more familiar with the variable picture of Lyme disease, and more knowledgeable about its treatment.

Testing for Lyme Disease

Testing for Lyme disease involves drawing blood and sending it to a lab to check for antibodies to the spirochete that causes this disease, using a sequential two-step process.[19] The most reliable results are usually achieved in those who are tested a few weeks to a month after infection — waiting less time may result in false negatives. Test results are usually available in a matter of weeks. It is also important to think about your risk factors. More than three-quarters of reported tickborne illness occurs in the southern-New-England and mid-Atlantic states, where white-tail deer — a frequent vector — are so plentiful as to be a nuisance.[20] Lyme disease is also found in the upper-Midwest states of Michigan, Minnesota, and Wisconsin, and in the Pacific states of California, Washington, and Oregon, where the danger of infection may be seasonal (limited to the spring months).[21] Doctors practicing in other areas of the country may not think to look for Lyme. However, you can usually find a Lyme disease specialist if you need one.

Treating Lyme Disease

Treating Lyme disease involves the use of oral antibiotics. They usually need to be taken for many months or even longer, so developing gut dysbiosis and candida overgrowth is a possibility. Make sure this is considered in your doctor's treatment plan. Sometimes, if the disease has progressed, intravenous antibiotics may be necessary, especially if symptoms are severe.[22]

Another important factor is the possibility of coinfection with other organisms. *Bartonella* spp., *Babesia* sp., and *Anaplasma* sp. are all tick-borne intracellular pathogens that can establish long-term, persistent infection with nonspecific symptoms.[23] In surveys of deer ticks in New Jersey, *Bartonella* (another tick-associated pathogen) was found to be as common, if not more common, than *Borrelia burgdorferi*, the organism that causes Lyme disease.[24] This is a specific area of study well beyond the scope of this book, but if you have a history of Lyme disease and your symptoms persist after treatment, another tick-borne infection should be suspected and, theoretically, treated with antibiotics.

However, some researchers and physicians feel that, based on the results of five double-blind clinical studies, antibiotic treatment of post-Lyme-disease symptoms is "not in the best interest of patients."[25] Whatever course of treatment you undertake, if any, should begin after a thorough discussion with a Lyme disease specialist, who also understands the chronic pain or chronic bladder symptoms you are experiencing.

If problems persist and any of the Lyme disease information presented here sounds vaguely familiar, check with your physician and ask to be tested.

Candida Overgrowth

Could an overgrowth of naturally occurring yeast be contributing to your urological symptoms? Many women have reported success in relieving their bladder symptoms after undergoing treatment for an overgrowth of the naturally occurring yeast *Candida albicans* (see Laura's story in Chapter 8). Candida can develop anywhere: in the mouth and throat (where it is called "thrush"), the gut, the vagina, the urethra, the skin under the breasts, and the skin around the anus. Yeast likes warmth and moisture, and it likes to not be interrupted — very similar to the conditions we give a loaf of bread to help it rise. *Candida albicans* is the species of yeast responsible for most yeast infections, but other infective strains of yeast exist, including *C. parapsilosis, C. tropicalis,* and *C. guilliermondii.*[26]

Yeast exists in balance with other organisms that make up our normal intestinal flora, but problems result when conditions in the body change to favor the proliferation of yeast, and the delicate balance is upset, a condition known as gut dysbiosis.

Many problems with yeast overgrowth are a result of elevated glucose levels from diabetes, from immune suppression due to illness, or from the use of immunosuppressant drugs or cancer treatments.[27] This is why many medical treatment plans should be geared to supporting overall health and the resolution of systemic conditions that favor yeast. Antibiotic therapy is one of the most favorable conditions under which yeast can proliferate. Other medications, including oral contraceptives, can increase the likelihood of vaginal yeast infections. Surgery, and viral infections that cause gastroenteritis, may also contribute to gut dysbiosis and candida overgrowth.

Symptoms

Symptoms caused by an overgrowth of candida include rashes, redness, skin irritation, itchiness, breakdown of pharyngeal (throat), oral, and esophageal mucosa, and vaginal symptoms such as white or yellowish discharge, odor, and discomfort. Unfortunately, candida can develop in the bladder, too, and even in the tiny urethral canal, causing irritation, burning, and a kind of annoying tickling that is torturous! This is why you will need the help of your urologist or gynecologist to prescribe a candida treatment concurrent with your long-term antibiotic treatment if you are diagnosed with an occult bacterial infection or with Lyme disease. More general symptoms may also include headaches, fatigue, sugar cravings, food allergies and intolerances, mental cloudiness or fogginess, and inflammation.

Diagnosis

Whether or not there is a need for a specific test for candida depends somewhat on which symptoms exist. Yeast is a normal component of the body's microorganisms, but it must exist in balance. Therefore, it is difficult to come up with a test able to distinguish candida overgrowth from normal yeast growth. Some doctors use a questionnaire covering a large array of yeast-related symptoms. A history of symptoms characteristic of candida overgrowth, such as skin rashes, fatigue, and mouth ulcers, along with a history of recurrent, recent, or long-term antibiotic use, is one clue that yeast overgrowth may be a problem. Some doctors may also look for antibodies that indicate the body is trying to fight off or suppress a yeast infection, but most people already have antibodies to candida. Other practitioners may examine a stool sample under the microscope to look for obvious candida. And if you have symptoms of oral or pharyngeal thrush — a white coating of yeast on the tongue and throat — a swab may be taken for culturing.

The best approach may be to work with your doctor to identify possible symptoms of candida, develop a diet plan for reducing candida over time, and keep track of your progress. Be forewarned: It isn't easy, and it can take a long time. But keep in mind that it is possible to have significant improvement of urogenital symptoms after treating for yeast overgrowth. If you have any of the risk factors we've discussed, perhaps this is your answer.

Controlling Candida

What can you do to help? If you are following a diet modified to exclude gluten, dairy, and sugar, you are already doing a great deal to make conditions less favorable for candida overgrowth. If you are currently experiencing problems with candida, you can further refine your diet to reduce all simple sugars, including those contained in sweet fruits, starchy vegetables, and grains, and to avoid foods that may contain mold or that have undergone fermentation (vinegar, peanuts, soy sauce, and some processed meats and cheeses).

A typical candida treatment program consists of the steps "weed, seed, feed." This refers to the need to first treat fungal infections with medications or an herbal approach ("weed"), followed by taking probiotics to restore beneficial microorganisms ("seed"), and the last step, transforming your diet to one that does not support the growth of candida, but instead supports the growth of beneficial gut bacteria ("feed"). These steps will be discussed in greater detail later in this chapter.

A visit to a naturopath may be in order. The naturopath will likely prescribe natural herbal antifungal treatments, but if your condition is severe enough, it may warrant treatment with systemic antifungals like Diflucan, or another antifungal drug like nystatin. Many traditional physicians prefer to use nystatin because when taken orally it isn't absorbed by the body but rather exerts its effect locally on the gastrointestinal tract through which it passes. Diflucan has the potential to cause liver toxicity in some individuals, but it is commonly prescribed in a limited dose for a prescribed period of time.

In addition, it is extremely important to treat gut dysbiosis by restoring the proper balance of microorganisms that are beneficial to the gut. These include strains of lactobaccillus and other beneficial bacteria that help to control the overgrowth of pathogenic bacteria and yeast. Some fermented foods like yogurt, kefir, sauerkraut, and miso (which contain live cultures), as well as regular use of high-quality probiotic supplements, can help a great deal. However, it is even more important to stop eating the sugars and simple carbohydrates on which yeast thrives. This is the philosophy behind the anti-candida diets prescribed by Dr. William Crook and many others (see Resources). Another benefit to an anticandida diet is that it is typically free of most grains, so you may have the added benefit of avoiding gluten as well.

The following antifungal herbs may be effective against candida, but they should only be used under the direction of a qualified herbalist, as they are very powerful and can have some toxicity if overused: golden seal, grapefruit-seed extract, pau d'arco, barberry, Oregon-grape root, echinacea, garlic, black walnut, caprylic acid (derived from coconut), and thyme. Drinking ginger tea or taking ½ teaspoon of cinnamon daily may also help to combat yeast. There are also many combination products for combating yeast overgrowth. Check with your natural pharmacy or consult with a naturopathic physician.

So what happens when you treat the yeast? It begins to die off and, as it does so, it releases toxins that can cause very uncomfortable symptoms including headaches, muscle aches, flulike chills, and nausea, to the point that some people feel temporarily worse. You can ease these sorts of symptoms by going more slowly on your program to combat yeast, and you may feel better by increasing your intake of liquids, taking warm baths, and adding yogurt and kefir to your diet.

What You Can Do Now

In this chapter, we've examined three of the "most likely suspects" regarding possible microorganisms that may be contributing to your bladder problems. If you have been ill for a long time and nothing seems to help, it is a good idea to take the time to thoroughly investigate each one and eliminate it as a possible cause of your symptoms. Of course, there is an expense involved, but this must be weighed against living indefinitely with a chronic illness. Alternatively, the right treatment could lead to living a life of wellness, free of chronic bladder pain, and the associated muscle aches, body pain, and fatigue that are common in IC and related illnesses. Anecdotally, women with lingering IC symptoms, despite a variety of allopathic treatments, have sometimes made good progress toward recovery by discovering a pathogenic source for their illness. Obtaining a urine broth culture or having testing done to rule out Lyme disease may be a very small price to pay to begin turning things around for you. Likewise, diagnosing and treating for candida overgrowth may pay big dividends.

11

Medical Conditions and Other Sources of Pelvic Pain or Bladder Symptoms

There are additional medical conditions that could be contributing to your pelvic pain or bladder symptoms, and, in fact, these may co-exist with IC and/or pelvic floor dysfunction (PFD). Some, like endometriosis, are well known, others are less familiar, and some are very serious. I've included this chapter in an effort to leave no stone unturned in your search for relief from chronic pelvic pain (CPP) and bladder symptoms.

Diabetes Mellitus

Many people are aware that urinary frequency and the voiding of large amounts of urine are common signs of diabetes. The most common type of diabetes, type II, occurs in adults and seniors, so when these symptoms begin to occur it may be a good idea to rule out diabetes as a possible cause rather than attributing them to overactive bladder or simply aging. It is easy to do this by visiting your medical practitioner for a checkup that includes some simple blood work.

In the medical text *Voiding Dysfunction: Diagnosis and Treatment*, author Dr. Rodney A. Appell discusses urological symptoms in diabetes. Although a significant number of patients initially have symptoms such as urinary frequency (78 percent), urgency, and nocturia (87 percent), more than half eventually develop a combination of neurogenic urological symptoms, including incomplete emptying, urinary hesitancy, and decreased stream flow.[1]

Diabetes mellitus, sometimes abbreviated DM, is fairly common, affecting approximately 8 to 9 percent of the general population, or nearly 24 million people in the United States. An estimated 5.7 million people with diabetes are undiagnosed.[2] There are two primary types of diabetes. Type I, or insulin-dependent diabetes, is caused by a complete failure of the pancreas to produce insulin, a hormone that enables the body to metabolize glucose, a simple form of sugar that the body uses for fuel. The age of onset varies from early childhood through young adulthood (it has previously been referred to as juvenile diabetes), and it is thought to be caused by a combination of hereditary factors and the body's autoimmune response to a virus or other immune-system dysfunction. There is a strong link between type I diabetes and celiac disease (hereditary gluten intolerance), and there may be triggers, such as the Epstein-Barr virus, which also causes mononucleosis. Simply put, in type I diabetes, the body attacks the pancreas and destroys its insulin-producing cells. Insulin must be supplied for life through subcutaneous shots or an implanted insulin pump. About 5–10 percent of all diabetics have type I diabetes.

Type II diabetes, or non–insulin-dependent diabetes, is caused by the body's developing either "insulin resistance," an inability to properly and efficiently metabolize glucose, or "insulin deficiency," a failure to produce enough insulin to meet the body's needs. The body usually continues to produce *some* insulin, so type II diabetes can often be treated through dietary and lifestyle changes, such as losing weight, regular exercise, and following a strict diabetic diet. Type II diabetes risk is inherited, and it is more common in some ethnic groups, including African-Americans, Hispanics, and Native Americans.

Age is also a risk factor for type II diabetes, and we are seeing more cases of it as the U.S. population ages. About 90 percent of people with diabetes have type II diabetes, and due to the obesity epidemic in our country, it is unfortunately becoming even more common and occurring in younger people than in the past.

Normal fasting morning glucose levels in adults are about 70–100 mg/dl (milligrams per deciliter), although there are some physicians who believe keeping fasting blood sugar under 90 is healthier. When our blood sugar is lower or significantly higher than this, especially for a sustained period, we can experience uncomfortable and even life-threatening symptoms. Sugar provides our brains and bodies with fuel, and what we cannot use immediately is stored in the liver. In diabetes, this system does not function normally. Our metabolic function is no longer on autopilot.

When we have too much glucose in the bloodstream — either because we've consumed more simple sugars than the body can process, because our pancreas is incapable of producing sufficient insulin, or because we've developed insulin resistance — we can experience symptoms of "hyperglycemia," or high blood sugar.

Symptoms of Hyperglycemia, or High Blood Sugar

Symptoms of hyperglycemia include the following:

- increased thirst
- increased urination (amount and frequency)
- increased drowsiness
- poor wound healing
- vision problems, such as blurred vision
- frequent opportunistic infections like yeast infections in skin folds, and increased incidence of urinary tract infections (UTIs)

In contrast, hypoglycemia, or low blood sugar, can occur in diabetics as a result of too much insulin or medication, vomiting, refusing meals after receiving insulin or medication, or due to another illness. It is important to note that hypoglycemia can also occur in people who are *not* diabetic. Hypoglycemia places a major strain on the adrenals, and it should be avoided or addressed during any program of adrenal recovery — by eating small, frequent meals, and avoiding sugar, simple carbohydrates, and other foods that contribute to hypoglycemia by stimulating the pancreas to produce too much insulin (in people who do not have diabetes).

Symptoms of Hypoglycemia, or Low Blood Sugar

Symptoms of hypoglycemia include the following:

- weakness and confusion
- hunger
- shakiness
- pale color
- moist, clammy skin

- anxiety
- light-headedness
- headache
- seizure
- coma

What about gestational diabetes? This type of diabetes, which develops during pregnancy (gestation), strains the body's ability to metabolize glucose. Gestational diabetes is considered a risk factor for developing type II diabetes later in life.

If you have a family history of diabetes, a personal history of gestational diabetes, borderline elevated glucose levels, are overweight, or experience any of the symptoms listed above, you should be evaluated by your physician for diabetes. Don't simply assume that your frequent urination needs to be treated symptomatically; it *could* be a symptom of a more serious disease, like diabetes.

Pelvic Endometriosis, Bladder Endometriosis, and Adenomyosis

Many of us know that endometriosis can cause bloating, tenderness, pain, swelling, and cramping in conjunction with monthly menstrual cycles. Here I'll give a thorough explanation, especially of the ways in which endometriosis can cause pelvic pain and bladder symptoms.

Pelvic Endometriosis

Approximately 10–35 percent (estimates vary greatly) of reproductive-age women have endometriosis, making it the most commonly reported cause of CPP.[3] In fact, a 2006 study showed that 83 percent of women with CPP who sought treatment at a center for pelvic pain were found to have active endometriosis upon laparoscopy (a minimally invasive procedure used to view the inside of the abdomen or pelvic cavity via a thin, flexible "endoscope" equipped with a camera).[4]

Endometrial cells make up the lining of the uterus. Endometriosis occurs when endometrial cells migrate from the interior of the uterus into the abdominal cavity, where they do not belong. This happens through a process known as "retrograde menstruation," in which endometrial cells flow from the uterus back through the fallopian tubes into the pelvic cavity, where they grow into clusters of endometrial tissue.[5] It is possible that this happens as a result of pelvic anatomy, or that it takes place during inverted exercises or yoga positions, or during sexual intercourse while menstruating, or it could be due to other unknown causes. Endometrial tissue in the pelvic cavity is hormonally sensitive; it swells and bleeds in conjunction with the monthly hormonal cycle, just like the endometrial tissue lining the uterus. This creates the cyclical fluctuations in pain, tenderness, and bloating characteristic of endometriosis. Endometrial tissue can settle on the ovaries, on the external surface of the uterus or bladder, and, in rare circumstances (less than 2 percent), on the inside of the bladder, a condition known as bladder endometriosis (see below).

The onset of pain from endometriosis often begins about a week prior to menstruation, peaks on the first day, and lasts another two or three days;[6] this cycle tends to be repeated on a monthly basis. That can mean eight to ten days each month of nearly constant pain!

How does pelvic endometriosis affect the bladder? Pelvic inflammation from endometriosis can put pressure on an already-sensitive bladder, greatly increasing urinary urgency and frequency. Hormonal fluctuations in the menstrual cycle can also increase inflammation, pain, and tenderness in the bladder itself, especially if endometrial cysts or tissue are present on either the external or (rarely) the internal surface of the bladder.

Bladder Endometriosis

Estimates of bladder endometriosis range from less than 2 percent to "relatively common," but most researchers agree that endometrial tissue is more often found on the outside of the bladder rather than on the internal surface.[7] When bladder endometriosis exists, symptoms include discomfort, pain or burning with urination, painful intercourse, blood in the urine, bladder tenderness, urinary frequency, urinary urgency, and sometimes urine retention.[8] Bladder endometriosis can be mistaken for a simple UTI, but urine cultures are usually negative.

One of the most important facts regarding bladder endometriosis is that it shares many of the same symptoms as IC. More than 70 percent of patients diagnosed with bladder endometriosis reported symptoms *identical* to those of IC.[9]

Many IC patients and many endometriosis patients share a history of irritable bowel syndrome (IBS), allergies, and migraines, as well as a family history of their respective diseases. This leads some researchers to suspect that a hereditary immunodeficiency or autoimmune process may be involved in these conditions.[10] A study reported in 2002 showed an increased incidence of autoimmune diseases in women with endometriosis. Specifically, there was an increased prevalence of lupus, multiple sclerosis (MS), rheumatoid arthritis, autoimmune hypothyroidism, Sjögren's syndrome, fibromyalgia, and asthma. Coincidentally, or not, this list is *identical* to the autoimmune disorders clinically associated with gluten intolerance and celiac disease.

Endometriosis can be diagnosed with a laparoscopy, during which the doctor performs biopsies (removal of tissue samples for examination under a microscope). A transvaginal ultrasound is also a useful and effective tool for diagnosing endometriosis of the bladder or ovaries, and it isn't nearly as uncomfortable as it sounds.[11]

Allopathic (i.e., traditional Western) medicine may offer birth control pills and other drug-based treatments to shrink endometrial tissue. In severe cases of bladder endometriosis, doctors may need to remove endometrial tissue surgically, or even perform a hysterectomy, a partial cystectomy, or both.

Some doctors try to manage mild to moderate endometriosis with hormone therapies or medications such as Lupron, which can shrink endometrial lesions and tissue, and is sometimes used to decrease the size of endometrial masses prior to surgery. However, Lupron has some significant drawbacks: it is very expensive, can cause permanent side effects in some people, and does not actually destroy the endometrial lesions that cause endometriosis.[12]

Some complementary-medicine practitioners have had success treating endometriosis by placing their patients on an organic diet

that also excludes meat, dairy, or poultry products containing hormones.[13] Avoiding the phytoestrogens found in soy may also help
some women with endometriosis. Acupuncture and other complementary pain treatments may be useful.

Endometriosis does not occur in females who have not yet begun to menstruate, and symptoms in older women generally begin to
fade with menopause. It is also important to know that endometriosis is a common cause of infertility: Twenty percent of women with
endometriosis are infertile.[14]

Adenomyosis

Adenomyosis is endometriosis of the uterus. But isn't the uterus a
normal place for endometrial tissue to grow? Yes, but this particular
condition results from an overgrowth of endometrial tissue invading
the muscular wall of the uterus (myometrium). Mainly found in premenopausal women between ages thirty-five and fifty, adenomyosis can cause the uterus to become heavier and bulkier (though not
necessarily larger), and it can result in symptoms such as very painful periods with profuse bleeding and general pelvic pain. Profuse
monthly bleeding can, in turn, lead to iron-deficiency anemia. The
cause of adenomyosis has not been clearly identified, but it is possible
that estrogen dominance, which is common in this age group, may
be involved. After menopause, when the production of estrogen de-
clines, symptoms typically are less severe.

Adenomyosis is differentiated from uterine fibroids because it
has a more diffuse pattern, in comparison to the well-defined mass
of a fibroid. Although transvaginal ultrasound is the most widely
available and economical diagnostic tool, MRI may be better able
to distinguish adenomyosis from multiple fibroid growths. MRI is
also useful for determining the depth of endometrial growth into
the uterine wall, which can aid the doctor in developing a treatment
plan.

Treatment options can include medications for pain and hormonal suppression, but the only permanent cure at this point is hysterectomy (removal of the uterus). Endometrial ablation (when an
overgrowth of cells in the uterine lining is destroyed or "ablated" by
the application of heat), while useful in other conditions affecting the

uterine lining, isn't useful in adenomyosis because the growth is not limited to the surface but has already penetrated the muscular wall. Although hysterectomy may not be an option you want to consider, it is worth discussing with your ob-gyn. Newer, less-invasive hysterectomies, involving more rapid recovery time, have been developed in recent years. Some of these are done vaginally and do not leave an exterior scar. In other types of hysterectomy, you may be able to keep your cervix, which can help maintain structural support within the pelvis. You may also elect to keep your ovaries if other conditions, such as endometriosis, have been ruled out by your physician. Discuss your treatment options with your doctor.

Although adenomyosis is a painful disorder that can greatly impact the lives of women who suffer from it, it does not appear to increase the risk of developing uterine cancer.

Chronic pelvic pain usually has more than one cause, and any of the three varieties of endometriosis discussed here may need to be ruled out as contributing to your symptoms. *It is important to remember that not all of your pelvic pain may be coming from within your bladder.* Pelvic adhesions, discussed next, are another possible source of chronic pelvic pain.

Pelvic Adhesions

Pelvic adhesions can develop when scar tissue or endometrial tissue forms bands that fuse organs together or wrap around sections of the bowel, ovaries, or fallopian tubes. Ordinarily, organs have some freedom of movement, which allows for bending, stretching, weight gain, growth of a fetus, and periodic fluctuations caused by hormones and fluid balance. Endometrial tissue can form adhesions between organs that restrict this freedom of movement, causing pain, infertility, discomfort with sexual intercourse, and other symptoms associated with moderate to severe cases of endometriosis.

In addition to endometrial tissue, adhesions also develop from scar tissue associated with trauma or injury to the pelvic and abdominal areas. Some of the possible causes of scar tissue adhesions include infection, chemotherapy, radiation, and cancer. However, by far the most common cause of pelvic adhesions is the development of scar tissue following abdominal and pelvic surgeries, one of the possible negative consequences of both cesarean deliveries and hysterectomies.[15]

In a study reported in 1997, 60–70 percent of all cases of small-bowel obstruction involved adhesions.[16] The impact of adhesions as a complication of abdominal and pelvic surgery is huge: Hundreds of thousands of surgeries are performed annually in the United States for removal of adhesions![17] Adhesions can cause chronic pelvic pain by constraining organs and tissues and by causing nerve entrapment. If the bowel becomes obstructed by a pelvic adhesion that encircles it, distention and gas will cause pain; this kind of pain alone will usually send people to the hospital, but other symptoms to recognize are nausea, vomiting, and a cessation of bowel movements. An obstructed bowel is life-threatening without prompt medical treatment. If you have ever had abdominal or pelvic surgery and are now suffering from bowel symptoms or chronic pelvic pain, ask your physician for a thorough evaluation to rule out the possibility of adhesions.

Pelvic Congestion

Pelvic congestion is an important cause of chronic pelvic pain usually confined to women who have undergone pregnancy and childbirth one or more times. It is caused by a weakening and dilation of the pelvic veins, similar to the development of varicose veins in the legs, which many women with pelvic congestion also have.

Symptoms can be mild or quite painful, and they tend to worsen over the course of the day, especially with prolonged sitting or standing. Pain can be experienced in the pelvic organs, and, frequently, in the vulva. Unlike many other types of chronic pelvic pain, the discomfort from pelvic congestion is described as a feeling of pressure, or a dull aching or "throbbing," which makes sense with a vascular disorder.

Pelvic venography, a procedure in which contrast dye is injected in order to better visualize the distended pelvic veins, is thought to be the best method of diagnosis. A transvaginal ultrasound may be useful in diagnosing this disorder, but pelvic congestion may be difficult to detect unless this test is performed when the patient is standing. (Lying down assists venous return, so sometimes tests done when the patient is lying down yield little useful information.)

Once properly diagnosed, a referral to an interventional radiologist is appropriate. There are successful options available for treating the distended veins that cause pelvic congestion, including embolization, a minimally invasive procedure involving only a short recovery period.

Ovarian Cysts

An ovarian cyst is a collection of fluid surrounded by a thin wall — similar in structure to a large blister — found within an ovary. It develops from an ovarian follicle, usually during ovulation, when the follicle does not rupture in a normal manner to release its egg. In some cases, a cyst can be filled with blood; this is known as a hemorrhagic cyst. If a hemorrhagic cyst ruptures, it releases blood into the pelvic cavity, creating irritation or pain.

Ovarian cysts are relatively common; many women experience at least one in their lifetime. In a diagnostic study conducted in Sweden, ovarian cysts were found in 6.6 percent of women ages twenty-five to forty.[18] Most of these types of cysts are benign, although some can grow to be quite large. Years ago, a woman in my Lamaze class had a softball-size ovarian cyst that was discovered during a routine ultrasound of her fetus. She required a cesarean section and removal of the cyst, because it would have prevented a safe vaginal delivery.

Most cysts arise spontaneously and resolve the same way. This is why your doctor may initially suggest conservative treatment. In a study of seventy women with cysts on one or both ovaries, patients were divided into four treatment groups. A control group received no medication or hormonal treatment. The other three groups received either oral contraceptives or other medications. At the six-week follow-up, complete resolution of cysts had occurred in two thirds (66 percent) of the control group but in only 53.9 to 57 percent of women in the treatment groups.[19] In another study, 82 percent of cysts in women ages twenty-five to forty resolved spontaneously after three months without any specific treatment.[20]

Ovarian cysts often cause mid-cycle pain that is located on only one side. Pain may come in mild twinges, or it can be severe. The pain of a right-sided ovarian cyst can be mistaken for appendicitis, but blood tests and CAT scans help to rule out this condition. Ovarian cysts can grow so large that they put pressure on the bladder, causing extreme urgency, frequency, and pain when the bladder is even partially full. For those with IC, this pain and pressure can be truly unbearable, and I speak from personal experience. Sometimes partial relief is experienced after the cyst ruptures and pressure on the bladder is relieved, but a ruptured cyst can also be very painful, especially a hemorrhagic cyst.

Women taking birth control pills don't produce ovarian cysts as often as those who are not on the pill, so this is one treatment your doctor may recommend if you suffer from repeated ovarian cysts. If necessary, an ob-gyn can evacuate, or draw the fluids out of, the cyst using a minor surgical procedure, but since most cysts resolve spontaneously, this is rarely done. Ovarian cysts impinging on the bladder can be easily visualized during a urodynamic fluoroscopy study.

Polycystic ovarian syndrome (PCOS) should be considered when ovaries contain multiple cystic follicles two to five millimeters in diameter. Your doctor will discuss this complicated disorder with you, as it involves many other symptoms and requires long-term management; a discussion of PCOS is beyond the scope of this book, but for anyone suffering from PCOS, I recommend reading *Positive Options for Polycystic Ovary Syndrome (PCOS)*, by Christine Craggs-Hinton and Adam Balen, MD.

Ovarian Cancer

A surprisingly large amount of information exists on the urological symptoms of ovarian cancer. Ovarian cancer is often caught too late for effective treatment, which leads to the unnecessary deaths of sixteen thousand women in the United States each year.[21] The disease affects one in a hundred women during their lifetime. The good news is that when detected early, ovarian cancer is very treatable, with a cure rate of 90 percent.[22] Unfortunately, early detection isn't common, which can make this rapidly growing cancer devastating.[23]

Risk of ovarian cancer increases with hormone exposure over one's lifetime. It is more likely to occur in women who are over forty (nine out of ten cases), have spent little or no time in pregnancy, have never taken contraceptives, have endometriosis, and have a family history of other gynecological cancers and breast cancer.

The most common symptom of ovarian cancer is crampy abdominal pain (not associated with diarrhea or vomiting) that lasts longer than two weeks. Other important symptoms can include the following:

- abdominal pressure, fullness, swelling, and bloating
- pelvic pain and pain with intercourse
- persistent indigestion, gas, nausea, and loss of appetite
- increased abdominal girth, resulting in clothes fitting tighter around the waist
- lower back pain

Early symptoms of ovarian cancer can be nonspecific and similar to symptoms of many other abdominal and pelvic conditions — and, as seen in the list above, not necessarily alarming. Other symptoms such as constipation, diarrhea, fatigue, and weight changes can also be important in diagnosing ovarian cancer. However, Barbara Goff, MD, professor and director of gynecologic oncology at the University of Washington, says, "Relatively new and persistent problems are the most important ones. So, the transient bloating that often accompanies menstrual periods would not qualify, nor would a lifelong history of indigestion."[24] It is very important to consider a change in pattern.

Importantly for those with chronic bladder issues, 18 percent of people in a 2004 Mayo Clinic study had urinary symptoms such as incontinence, urgency, and frequency that grew increasingly worse over a two- or three-week period.[25] This was an important and widely published study, because it was previously thought that only late signs of ovarian cancer were detectable, and now we know that it can cause symptoms at earlier stages.[26] Barbara Goff says, "The urinary problems reported in the study (urgency, frequency, worsening incontinence) were classic symptoms of bladder infections, which are common in women. But it still makes sense to consult a doctor, because bladder infections should be treated. Urinary trouble that persists despite treatment is a particular cause for concern."[27]

Urgency and frequency symptoms may also be associated with later stages of ovarian cancer, because the tumor may press on the bladder. Increased incidence of urinary tract infection may also result as tumors create blockages of the ureters. In later stages of ovarian cancer, these symptoms can be addressed surgically as part of palliative care, helping to make patients more comfortable.

Fewer than 25 percent of women with ovarian cancer report gynecological symptoms such as irregular menstruation.[28] However, bleeding after menopause, or during or after sexual intercourse, should not be considered normal and should be reported to your physician, as these may be signs of ovarian cancer.

In conclusion, the characteristic pattern doctors see most often in ovarian cancer is persistent and/or worsening symptoms. The Mayo Clinic study showed that in contrast to most digestive disorders, in which symptoms tend to come and go or are provoked by eating certain foods, there is less fluctuation with ovarian cancer. Symptoms are present all of the time, and they gradually become worse.[29]

Bladder Cancer

Although the possibility of bladder cancer is a nagging worry for many people who experience severe pain, hematuria (blood in the urine), and other frightening symptoms, bladder cancer is infrequent in women, and it is often linked to past or current exposure to nicotine, nitrates, industrial chemicals and dyes, pesticides, and other carcinogens. However, bladder cancer is more common in men. Studies in the United Kingdom showed ten thousand new cases of bladder cancer per year, three-quarters of which were in men, which translates to one in thirty men developing this cancer in their lifetime.[30] Bladder cancer is more common among whites than other ethnic groups and in men over forty (usually over fifty).[31] People whose work constantly exposes them to chemicals used in leather manufacture, hairdressing, and spray-painting are at high risk, especially when exposure lasts many years. Smoking, however, is the major known cause of bladder cancer; it is thought to cause up to half of all bladder cancers in men, and a third of bladder cancers in women. One of the best things smokers can do for their bladder and their overall health is to quit smoking.

Your physician can speak with you about your concerns and conduct tests to rule out the possibility of bladder cancer. Cystoscopy and biopsy are the only definitive tests, and patients with significant risk factors should insist on receiving them.[32] If you have a cystoscopy to look at the inside of your bladder in order to diagnose IC, bladder cancer is always one of the possibilities your doctor is looking for during the procedure. Keep in mind, though, that no evidence exists that IC/PBS increases the risk of bladder cancer.

The following is a list of common symptoms of bladder cancer:

- blood or blood clots in the urine (hematuria, which occurs in 80 to 90 percent of people who have bladder cancer and is the most common symptom)
- pain during urination (dysuria)
- urinating small amounts frequently and, in general, experiencing urgency and frequency
- frequent UTIs (note that this usually isn't the case with IC)

Symptoms that may indicate more advanced bladder cancer include the following:

- bladder pain and abdominal pain
- pain in the lower back around the kidneys, sometimes radiating to the sides of the torso
- swelling in the lower legs
- a growth in the pelvis near the bladder (pelvic mass)

Other symptoms that could develop when bladder cancer has spread include the following:

- weight loss
- bone pain, or pain in the rectal, anal, or pelvic area
- anemia

The symptoms of bladder cancer can be similar to symptoms of more common bladder conditions, including UTI, but 25 percent of patients with bladder cancer have *no* reported symptoms.[33] Pay attention to or, better yet, avoid known risk factors such as smoking and chronic chemical exposure.

Other Conditions

This last section discusses some of the more remote possibilities that can be explored in an effort to track down the source of your bladder problems. Neurological damage resulting from trauma or other sources is included in this discussion.

Disk Problems

Irritation of the nerves in the lower back and sacrum resulting from a back injury, auto accident, degenerative disc disease, or sciatica can sometimes cause symptoms in the pelvis. These might include urinary frequency; irregular pain, numbness, or tingling in the back of the legs, buttocks, thighs, or rectum; and, in some cases, testicular pain in men. However, symptoms characteristic of many other common bladder disorders, such as burning with urination, hematuria, or a feeling of unbearable pressure in the bladder, are typically *not* present. An MRI can show your physician whether the discs in your lower back are pressing on your nerves, possibly causing your symptoms.

Multiple Sclerosis (MS)

Multiple sclerosis, or MS, is an autoimmune disease in which the protective myelin sheath that surrounds the nerves is gradually destroyed. It has a typical age of onset between thirty and fifty, and it affects more females than males by a ratio of three to one. MS is characterized by neurological symptoms that follow a pattern of worsening and then sometimes remission, and include vision problems, weakness of the extremities, and bladder dysfunction. Urinary symptoms are common, eventually affecting 50–80 percent of patients surveyed in clinical studies. In fact, a 1995 study of more than two hundred patients concluded that nearly every MS patient exhibits some degree of lower urinary tract abnormality, regardless of the state of progression of their disease.[34] These symptoms also follow a pattern of remission and exacerbation.[35] MS-related urological symptoms are associated with instability of the detrusor muscle (part of the bladder wall musculature — see Chapter 2), and they typically fall under the following categories:

- **symptoms of storage dysfunction:** urinary frequency, urgency, incontinence, nocturia, and pain — associated with hyperactivity (increased responsiveness) of the detrusor muscle

- **symptoms of emptying dysfunction:** hesitancy, difficulty starting a stream of urine, and incomplete emptying — associated with hypoactivity (decreased responsiveness) of the detrusor muscle

- **symptoms of both storage and emptying dysfunction** — associated with variable responsiveness and activity of the detrusor muscle

The most important goal in managing urinary problems in MS patients is to help them control their symptoms, sometimes by making changes, such as scheduled voiding.[36] Because MS often follows a degenerative pattern, some patients eventually develop a condition called "neurogenic bladder"; they may need to be catheterized or employ other long-term interventions.

What You Can Do Now

See your physician if you would like to be evaluated for any of these disorders. You will then need a referral to a specialist, as these disorders are seldom treated by a urologist or ob-gyn — yet another reason why obtaining an accurate diagnosis is crucial. If you are still searching for an accurate diagnosis or feel that you've been misdiagnosed, it never hurts to have your primary-care doctor take another look at your overall health. Reviewing these disorders illustrates that not all bladder and pelvic symptoms are generated within the bladder, or even within the pelvis. Our bodies can seem surprisingly mysterious until there is a "shift" in the way we view certain symptoms and behaviors, and then sometimes the answer becomes clear.

12

Some Effective Complementary Therapeutic Techniques

A valuable way to promote healing is to take advantage of techniques that balance and energize the body's vital organs and systems. This chapter describes three such therapies, but there are many others to choose from. It is always useful to obtain a personal recommendation when choosing any health practitioner. Also, remember to ask any complementary health practitioners you visit if they accept medical insurance. More practitioners are beginning to do so, and more insurance plans are offering complementary-medicine coverage.

Neurofascial Processing (NFP)

I actively resisted learning the technique known as NFP, regarding it as something I didn't think could possibly work—until I needed it. Although my complementary practitioner had introduced me to NFP and urged me for several years to practice it regularly, I really didn't give it much thought, and certainly not much effort. However, at one point I found myself in severe pain while backpacking in a remote desert area, and I had to call on all the tools at my disposal. I remembered NFP, tried it—and it worked. I tried it again—and it worked. Now I think of NFP as first aid for the body, via the body.

NFP is a simple, easy-to-learn technique that can contribute to improved health in several ways. To understand how it works, think of the body as containing a big electrical grid, with many substations controlling power output and storage. When one area has a large demand, the other areas in the grid can expand (or release energy) to meet that demand.

According to NFP, the body's major neurofascial processing centers are the following:

- the motor cortex of the brain (top of the head)
- the frontal lobes of the brain (behind the forehead)
- the limbic system of the brain (bridge of the nose)
- the thyroid (front of the throat)
- the heart
- the lungs (both front and back sides of the torso)
- the spleen (left side of the abdomen)
- the liver (right side of the abdomen)
- the pancreas (central upper abdomen)
- the kidneys (mid-back)
- the ureters (low back)
- the uterus (central pelvic area); the prostate is the corresponding center in men
- the upper and lower arms

In Western medicine these processing centers correspond to different organ systems; in Eastern medicine they correspond to the chakras. In addition to these major processing centers, secondary processing centers are located in the eyes, hands, knees, and feet.

Some of the processing centers are specific for certain actions. The ureters, for example, help the body rid itself of toxins and inflammation, and they are also useful for treating any area that is experiencing pain. The heart and the limbic centers also have the ability to help alleviate pain.

NFP can be used to treat specific conditions quickly, such as headache or middle-of-the-night bladder pain. In addition, for the long term, regularly connecting the processing centers during a quiet time of the day or evening helps to strengthen each system of the body and improve the communication between systems. I have used NFP to alleviate a variety of problems, including migraine headaches associated with my menstrual cycle, tension headaches, and bladder spasms.

So, how do you practice NFP? You can simply connect any two processing centers by placing a hand over each one and holding the position as long as you comfortably can, ideally for twenty minutes. To connect hard-to-reach areas, such as the ureters, which are located in the small of the back, you may need to invert your hand position, placing the back of the hand over the area rather than the palm. You can also connect a processing center with an area of injury, pain, or inflammation — the heart or the ureters are great "first aid" processing centers. Simply place one hand over your heart (or ureters) and the other on the area of injury or pain. I've observed that the more often I perform a specific NFP connection, the deeper and quicker the response, so practicing often is a good thing to do. It is also very helpful to take a course offered by a health professional or work with one privately to learn more about this useful technique.

I know NFP sounds unlikely and a little odd, but practicing it is so easy and effective that it is definitely worth trying. Clothing does not restrict the process, and you can do it discreetly almost anywhere, anytime. Picture yourself sitting in a long business meeting, or on a car ride, and your bladder starts acting up. Choose either the ureters or liver as your processing center, and put your other hand discreetly over your lower abdomen. If you're at a conference table, no one would be able to see, and if they did, they might think you had some minor indigestion.

To learn more about NFP, work with a specially trained physical therapist or a practitioner of IMT, described below. For a complete description of the NFP process, refer to the book *Body Wisdom: Light Touch for Optimal Health*, by Dr. Sharon Weiselfish-Giammatteo, the woman who developed the technique.[1]

One last point about NFP: To me it is much simpler to learn and to do than Reiki, in which a practitioner promotes healing and relaxation by laying her or his hands on a patient's body to manipulate the flow of *ki*, the Japanese word for "life energy" (similar to the Chinese concept of *chi*). There really is very little training involved in NFP, and no certification is required. (That said, if you have access to a Reiki practitioner, by all means get as much of this healing and pain-relieving treatment as you can.) In addition, from personal experience and on the advice of many physical therapists, the Chinese movement technique known as *qi gong* (pronounced and sometimes spelled *chi kung*) is also very beneficial in learning to breathe properly, relaxing the pelvic floor, and strengthening posture and balance. It is much easier to learn and to perform than the more familiar "tai chi," and I believe it has real benefits in teaching us how to relax the pelvic floor, which in turn, will help to decrease bladder and pelvic pain.

Integrative Manual Therapy (IMT)

IMT, also developed by Dr. Sharon Weiselfish-Giammatteo, is a set of methods used to assess and treat pain, dysfunction, and disease. IMT achieves healing through the skill of uniquely trained practitioners who work with the body's motilities, or natural biological rhythms. According to official descriptions of this technique, IMT practitioners are trained to eliminate protective recovery motilities and reset normal patterns, with a goal of helping the body achieve stability of its natural rhythms. IMT was developed in the 1970s and has a good track record of successful treatment, especially in difficult-to-treat cases. (Craniosacral therapy, which also works with the body's natural rhythms, may be more familiar.) IMT has sought to further develop this practice of working with the body's natural rhythms.

A typical session begins with the patient standing while the practitioner assesses posture and flexibility in the spine and upper body. The client is then asked to lie on a comfortable massage table. The IMT practitioner uses specially honed senses of touch and visualization to feel the body's rhythms. Unlike Reiki, IMT does not involve energy healing or any transfer of energy from or through the practitioner to the client. IMT practitioners use a light, gentle touch and frequently they will keep their hands in one location for several minutes until they can feel the change in pattern that needs to take place. The patient may feel very relaxed, and also may feel something shift, or become "unstuck." Drinking a glass of water following a session is recommended. If a patient has a significant amount of inflammation, he or she may void more urine than usual afterward as things begin to move in the lymphatic and urological systems.

While I make no claim of truly understanding IMT as a practice, I have been receiving great benefit from it for a number of years. In February of 2005 I began to experience very frequent pain in my upper back, neck, and trapezius (the muscle just above the collar bone that connects the head and shoulder). The pain worsened throughout the day, precipitating a one-sided migraine at the back of my head. The problem may have been the result of an old nursing-related musculoskeletal injury. Over the next few months, the pain became chronic; by August it was a daily occurrence. It was very severe. Each afternoon I became incapacitated by terrible migraines that affected my sensory system, caused nausea and intractable pain, and made it impossible for me to live a normal life. I sought help from general practitioners, headache specialists, chiropractors, and osteopaths, but got very little relief. The first time I experienced significant relief was following a session of craniosacral therapy, after which I was headache-free for four days. I knew I was on the right track, and I began to receive regular craniosacral sessions, but the longest period of relief I had was a week, at best. I researched nerve blocks, and over the next few months I had many weeks of relief but never a true healing. I was stuck in a pattern that the nerve blocks only impeded, and when they wore off, the headaches and back, neck, and trapezius pain returned.

Finally, in November of 2006 I had an appointment with a very skilled IMT practitioner. Afterward, my head still hurt, but my trapezius was much more relaxed. Something had changed, and gradually, over the next few days, the improvement continued. On the fourth day, I did not experience the familiar pattern of afternoon pain worsening into a migraine. I wondered how long the effect would last, but over time I forgot to think about it as I resumed my life after missing out on a big chunk of it for nearly two years. I did not have another migraine until July 2007, and, again, a single IMT session relieved the problem.

Like any of the medical arts, IMT depends on the knowledge and skill of the practitioner. (I'm very lucky to have one of the best!) My response isn't necessarily typical, and IMT isn't a miracle—but it is unique. It addresses the whole body in a gentle, noninvasive manner, and it can effect big changes in very little time. IMT is practiced by trained, licensed health practitioners, including some physical therapists, occupational therapists, massage therapists, nurses, osteopaths, and traditional medical doctors. It is billable under many insurance plans. For more information on IMT, please check out the websites listed in Resources.

One last word on IMT: It is very helpful in treating the symptoms of gluten intolerance and is particularly good at helping the bodies of sensitive individuals rid themselves of accumulated damage from gluten exposure. Regular IMT treatments have been instrumental in helping my body recover from undiagnosed celiac disease and from IC.

Acupuncture

Acupuncture is a two-thousand-year-old form of Chinese medicine. A practitioner makes use of very thin, almost hairlike needles inserted into specific points along the body's "meridians" to effect changes in the patient's energy level, pain level, immune system, and the function of various internal organs. It is usually not painful, although there may be mild discomfort at times. Overall, I would say it feels relaxing. Minor bruising can occur occasionally. It may be beneficial to include regular acupuncture treatments in your recovery plan, especially if you have access to a skilled acupuncturist. A common rule of thumb is: If you don't feel any improvement or relief in four or five treatments, then either the skill of the practitioner isn't adequate, or acupuncture isn't able to address your particular needs. This does not mean that you should be cured of all of your symptoms in four or five weeks of treatment; it simply means that you should have begun to feel *some* benefit or movement in the direction you want to go.

Not a lot of evidence exists in published literature regarding successful treatment of IC or CPP with acupuncture. However, a small study was conducted recently of patients in England who had failed to respond to conventional therapies such as medications, hydrodistention, and bladder instillations. Thirteen of the fifteen subjects demonstrated an improvement in symptoms and self-reported quality-of-life following only three sessions of acupuncture.[2] In 2004 and 2005 the University of Pennsylvania Pain Medicine Center was recruiting for a clinical study entitled "Acupuncture for the Treatment of Interstitial Cystitis (IC) Symptoms," but I am not aware of any published results from that study.[3]

Acupuncturists often prescribe Chinese herbs. Many of these herbs are meant to tone the bladder, and, therefore, they may be too powerful for the fragile IC bladder, which may already have an excess of muscle tone from frequent bladder spasms. If you choose to use Chinese herbs, I advise exercising a little caution. While there are many reports on the effectiveness of using Chinese herbs to treat asthma and other chronic ailments, my experience with Chinese herbs used to treat the bladder has not been positive.

Acupuncture may be very useful, though, in treating the frustrating and uncomfortable symptoms of menopause and in helping to balance cortisol levels in those suffering from chronic stress.[4] Many people find acupuncture to be relaxing and restorative, and they go on to make it an important part in regaining their health.

What You Can Do Now

NFP, IMT, Reiki, and acupuncture are just some of the mind-body healing arts you can seek out as part of your overall healing strategy. As I noted in my acknowledgements, it sometimes "takes a village" to help you begin to recover your health. Certainly, my recovery was aided by many gifted healers in a variety of complementary or "integrative" healing professions. If you are intuitively drawn to a particular healing art, then that is a good place to start. Ask your physician for referrals, but also ask close friends if they have any suggestions. There are abundant web listings for local resources and national professional groups in your area (see Resources). Avail yourself of the powerful effects of natural healing. It could make a big difference in your life. Yes, it can be costly, but it may be possible for you to attend a clinic or college of massage or acupuncture in your area. There is often a substantially reduced cost, and students are usually very closely supervised.

13

Other Helpful Diets to Consider

It should be obvious by now that following a specific diet plan may be the key to overall health and a return to bladder wellness for many people. We've discussed, in detail, the anti-inflammatory diet and the gluten-free diet in previous chapters. In this chapter you'll find the additional resources you need to change your diet as part of your overall self-treatment plan.

Introduction to Alternative Diets

Food is many things—fuel for our bodies and brains; nutrients necessary for growth, development, and the repair of damaged tissues; and a source of pleasure that nourishes our spirits. Food can also influence our bodies in other important ways. What we choose to eat can have powerful effects, including the following:

- contribute to or help alleviate inflammation
- affect our body's pH, or acid/alkaline balance, which has a great impact on our overall health and ability to recover from illness
- trigger allergic reactions and autoimmune responses, both of which have the potential to create bladder symptoms

I hope that you will take this opportunity to read through all of the diets described here, and to ask your physician if any of them could be applicable to your specific health needs. An important key to my recovery involved excluding all of the following: gluten, dairy, cane sugar, all sources of caffeine and, to a lesser extent, corn and soy. Your answer may be different. In addition to the gluten-free diet, outlined in Appendix A, information is provided in this chapter on several other diets, including a low-oxalate diet, a low-histamine diet, and the Body Ecology Diet, designed to heal a leaky intestinal lining, or "leaky gut." The chapter concludes with a guide to planning an "elimination diet," designed to methodically track down your individual food sensitivities.

Cultivating a Healthy Intestinal System: A Key to Recovering Your Health

Whichever dietary option you choose to follow, including your current diet, it is important to understand the role that probiotics, or the naturally occurring microorganisms that make up our intestinal flora, play in maintaining our health. Scientists who study the human gastrointestinal system have identified more than five thousand separate species of gut bacteria in normal human flora,[1] and I suspect this number will be discovered to be much higher with time. A strong, healthy gut flora, known as the human microbiome, enables the body to deal more effectively with "hitchhikers"—bacteria, viruses, and other microbes that we ingest along with our food— thus preventing gastrointestinal disease. These organisms also help break down plant material to make nutrients available and help in the manufacture and conversion of certain vitamins—especially vitamin K and the B vitamins. Healthy gut microbes also help to break down lectins (see Chapter 5), making our food more digestible and less likely to trigger immune reactivity. In fact, some scientists are discovering that food allergies and autoimmune disorders are far less common in cultures whose diets and lifestyles foster a healthy internal environment.[2] This is a new and exciting field of science with important implications for our future health!

From an allergy-prevention perspective, probiotics help the digestion process to break down proteins more thoroughly so that they cannot leak through the gut wall and create an allergenic response. Another critical role these beneficial organisms have is to help the body understand the boundary between self and nonself, which is essential for proper immune-system function. For all these reasons, it is a very good idea, whether ill or not, to take a probiotic regularly.

Some probiotics are packaged with FOS, or fructo-oligosaccharides, a particular type of "food" for gut organisms, to which some people are sensitive. Reactions range from experiencing excess gas to an increase in bladder pain.

Truly understanding the role of probiotics involves awareness of what happens when we take antibiotics. In clinical studies using standard dosing of Cipro (ciprofloxacin), a commonly prescribed antibiotic, one-third of all strains and species of gut bacteria were profoundly affected by only a five-day course.[3] Because the number of species and organisms is so large, some scientists feel that restoring our gut flora by ingesting probiotics is futile, and some clinical studies have shown a natural restoration of many gut bacteria species in as little as a few weeks. This may be the case for occasional or infrequent use of a single antibiotic. But what happens when you take long-term antibiotics, multiple antibiotics, daily prophylactic antibiotics, or frequent and repeated courses of antibiotics? Does the body really have the ability to restore itself from this kind of damage to its intestinal flora without assistance? Given the frequent history of infections with the pathogen *Clostridium difficile* following hospital-administered antibiotics, *Candida albicans* overgrowth, poor digestion, the development of multiple food sensitivities, allergies, and leaky gut syndrome, it appears that the answer is "probably not," at least in certain individuals. It is important to realize that we may need to assist in restoring helpful, naturally occurring organisms in order to keep the balance and prevent or control the growth of more harmful organisms that can cause serious illness. We do this by using over-the-counter probiotics and by eating a diet that supports our digestive health, such as the one described below.

The Body Ecology Diet (BED)

The BED was originally developed by Donna Gates to treat intestinal hyperpermeability, better known as "leaky gut," and it is described in her very popular book of that name, first published in 1996.[4] This diet recommends promoting healthy bacteria and enzymes by supplementing with naturally fermented products like kefir, yogurt, and naturally fermented or cultured vegetables like pickled cabbage (i.e., sauerkraut).[5] Like many of the best diets for improved health, the BED also drastically reduces the intake of simple carbohydrates and sugars, which feed *Candida albicans*, to the detriment of more beneficial microorganisms. The diet is useful for rebuilding immunity and is sometimes prescribed to treat chronic fatigue syndrome and other chronic illnesses. For more information, I recommend Donna Gates's website, www.bodyecology.com.

Leaky Gut Syndrome: A Case of Intestinal Hyperpermeability

The theory behind "leaky gut syndrome," or intestinal hyperpermeability, is that injury to and inflammation in the gastrointestinal tract can begin to break down the protective barrier of gut mucosa and lead to a variety of symptoms, from food allergies and intolerances, to gastrointestinal discomfort, to decreased immunity. This is because the naturally occurring "gaps" in the intestinal barrier, which are normally so small as to allow only foods digested down to essential nutritional components like amino acids and sugars to pass through into the bloodstream, are not functioning properly. When incompletely digested food particles leak into the bloodstream, this triggers the immune system to create inflammation and also triggers the development of food allergies. Theoretically, leaky gut syndrome can also lead to autoimmune reactions, either to the gastrointestinal tract, or to other areas in the body. This may be partially due to the fact that a major portion of the immune system is located in the gut itself, which makes sense, given the important role an intact and functional intestinal barrier plays in protecting us from potentially harmful microorganisms and toxins present in our food supply.

One of the keys to repairing a leaky gut is to correct the balance of our intestinal flora, and in the case of the BED diet, by taking specialized probiotics and cultured vegetables, and avoiding the foods that feed organisms common in gut dysbiosis, like *Candida albicans*.[6]

Related Diets

Two other diets to learn more about in your search for improved health are the Specific Carbohydrate Diet, developed by the late Elaine Gotschall, to aid in the treatment of IBS and detailed in the book *Breaking the Vicious Cycle*, and the Paleo diet, both of which limit grains and legumes and avoid all simple sugars.[7]

The Low-Oxalate Diet

Oxalates are found mostly in plant foods (in varying amounts), but they can also be found in lesser amounts in animal sources. In chemical terms, they are organic acids. Why may a low-oxalate diet be useful? There are several reasons, actually. Oxalates (also known as oxalic acid) have a natural affinity for binding up minerals from the digestive tract, making them unavailable for absorption. There are some rare health conditions, which I won't go into here, which require restriction of oxalates. From a urological perspective, oxalates, binding with calcium, are involved in the formation of the majority of kidney stones. Interestingly, some women who suffer from feminine discomfort and uncomfortable or painful intercourse (vulvodynia or vestibulitis) find that avoiding foods high in oxalates appears to help alleviate symptoms. Eating foods high in oxalates, on the other hand, often is reported to trigger or worsen symptoms. On this diet, foods are divided into three groups: low-oxalate foods with less than 2 mg of oxalate per serving, moderate-oxalate foods with 2–6 mg of oxalate per serving, and high-oxalate foods, which contain 7 or more mg per serving. To prevent calcium oxalate kidney stones, guidelines suggest staying below a total of 40–50 mg per day. To help prevent vulvodynia and vestibulitis symptoms, many women try to avoid all high-oxalate foods entirely, eat moderate-oxalate foods only occasionally, and form the bulk of their diets from low-oxalate foods.

Low-Oxalate Foods—Recommended

The following foods can be eaten freely on the low-oxalate diet:

- All meats, eggs, fish, poultry, dairy products (unflavored), fats and oils are low in oxalates and can be eaten freely.

- Low-oxalate vegetables include acorn and zucchini squashes, cabbage, cauliflower, iceberg lettuce, peas, and turnips.
- Low-oxalate fruits include apples, avocados, bananas, cantaloupe, honeydew, watermelon, sweet cherries, green grapes, nectarines, papayas, and mangoes. These can be eaten freely.
- White and wild rice are low-oxalate starches.

Moderate-Oxalate Foods—Eat Occasionally

Choose foods from this group for occasional use, perhaps two to three times per week, unless symptoms become aggravated:

- Moderate-oxalate vegetables include asparagus, artichokes, Brussels sprouts, carrots, broccoli, corn, cucumbers, lettuce, mushrooms, potatoes, and snow peas.
- Moderate-oxalate fruits and nuts include apricots, citrus fruits, peaches, pears, pineapple, plums, prunes, walnuts and almonds.
- Cornmeal-based products, brown rice, and oatmeal are moderate-oxalate starches.

As you can see, there is a fair amount of variety in a low- to moderate-oxalate diet. Now for the difficult part—below is a list of high-oxalate foods that may trigger vulvodynia and vestibulitis symptoms in some sensitive women.

High-Oxalate Foods—*Not* Recommended

The following high-oxalate foods may provoke symptoms in sensitive people, and they are not recommended if you suffer from frequent kidney stones or vulvodynia (pain in the vulva in women):

- Draft beer, chocolate, cocoa, coffee, black tea, pecans, cashews, walnuts, peanuts and peanut butter, dark-colored berries such as blueberries, blackberries, and black raspberries, rhubarb (very high!!!), wheat germ, and wheat-based baked goods.
- Many strongly flavored or bitter greens are very high in oxalates: beet greens, collards, dandelion, escarole, kale, leeks, mustard greens, parsley, parsnips, green peppers, spinach, sweet potatoes, yams, watercress, and sorrel.

- Spices and condiments high in oxalates include soy sauce, ginger, parsley, cinnamon, black pepper, and marmalade (and anything made with citrus peel).

- Legumes, including green beans, yellow wax beans, dried beans, baked beans, and soy products, including tofu, are all high in oxalates.

For a more complete list of oxalate levels in certain foods, abundant web sources exist. Two good ones are:

http://www.upmc.com/HealthAtoZ/Pages/HealthLibrary.aspx
    ?chunkiid=196214

http://www.proven-natural-medicine.com/oxalates.html

The Low-Histamine Diet

Foods containing histamine, or that cause the release of histamine from mast cells, can act as bladder irritants. The urine of people with IC has been found to contain elevated levels of histamine. Evidence also shows that many people with IC have found that their symptoms decrease when on an antihistamine, and antihistamines are commonly prescribed as part of an overall treatment plan. In addition to provoking IC symptoms, many of these foods can also trigger migraine headaches, which are also common in IC sufferers. Below are some lists of high-histamine foods that I have compiled from a variety of current sources.

High-Histamine Foods to Avoid

Bananas, chocolate, cranberries, raspberries, strawberries, pineapple, citrus, eggplant, pickles, pumpkin, sauerkraut, soy products, tomato products, raw egg whites, beef, chicken liver, pork, shellfish (scallops, shrimp), canned tuna fish, cheese, beer, red wine, yeast, foods containing yeast, and vinegars.

Sometimes sensitive people react to fish and seafood, and sometimes they don't. This may be because some foods, especially fish and seafood, produce histamines as they age from the conversion of naturally present histidine. If very freshly caught and frozen or eaten within a short time they may be tolerable, but at other times these same foods, when beginning to age, may provoke symptoms. In general, aged and fermented foods commonly have higher histamine levels. Histamine is heat-resistant and cannot be removed by cooking.[8]

Some people who are sensitive to histamines may also react to tartrazine and other food colorings, as well as preservatives including benzoates, sulfites, and BHA/BHT.[9] Accidentally eating foods containing either sulfites or potassium sorbate have, in the past, produced some of my worst bladder flares, so I do my best to avoid all processed foods, and I'm diligent about reading labels.

For more information on this topic, refer to the following websites:

http://www.urticaria.thunderworksinc.com/pages/lowhistam ine.htm. This site is provided by ICUS — the International Chronic Urticaria Society (urticaria refers to hives, a common symptom of an allergic reaction).

http://www.allergyuk.org/fs_histamine.aspx. This website for the British Allergy Foundation features a FAQ pdf that lists high-histamine foods.

Helpful Supplements for Those with Histamine Sensitivity

Vitamin C has an antihistamine effect, and, along with bioflavonoids that help moderate histamine release, can be helpful. Magnesium may also help to control histamine release. Nettle-leaf tea is a natural antihistamine, and it is useful to carry in a purse to use when travelling. Nettle-leaf tea is available as a bulk herb or in tea bags.

The Allergy Elimination Diet

Easy and effective, the allergy elimination diet requires dedication, but it produces highly individualized information on how your body reacts to specific foods. By beginning with the foods least likely to provoke a reaction, and then introducing new foods one-at-a-time, you will have a chance to notice any of the subtle — or not-so-subtle — ways in which your body responds. For example, you may be doing just fine, and then during the three days following the introduction of green peppers, you notice a lot more discomfort in your joints. Another food introduction may trigger a runny nose, a headache, or bladder spasms. Give the allergy elimination diet a serious try if you already suspect food sensitivities or if you suffer from poor health and don't know why. It is a very economical way to begin fine-tuning your diet to meet your body's individual needs. Another option is to have food allergy or sensitivity testing done by a qualified medical practitioner.

Getting Started

Here's how to start:

1. **Make up your daily diet of the following foods, and only these foods:**
   - *one protein* — start with salmon or lamb — if you don't eat red meat, turkey makes a good substitute; avoid the top allergens like shellfish, dairy products, eggs, and tree nuts
   - *one fruit* — start with pears, the least allergenic fruit — avoid top allergens like citrus and some berries
   - *one vegetable* — start with carrots, iceberg lettuce, or jicama, a very good vegetable for the bladder (although spinach, one of the least allergenic vegetables, is traditional, it isn't a good choice for those with IC or vulvodynia, as it is high in oxalates)
   - *one grain* — start with white rice; although it is less nutritious, it is slightly less likely to produce an allergic reaction than brown rice due to its lower protein content
   - *one oil or fat* — start with coconut oil or olive oil; for now, avoid nut oils, especially peanut oil
   - *sea salt*

2. **Eat only these foods for three days.** Vegetables and fruits may cooked, raw, or juiced. Rice can be rice cereal, cooked rice, rice milk (as pure as possible, and without sugar). Salmon or lamb should be broiled with a little sea salt and a little olive oil, if necessary. You can eat as much as you want or need to of any of these food choices, in any form desired. Just avoid introducing any new food items until you're sure you can tolerate these.

3. **Keep a record of how you feel during these three days,** how
   you slept, and what symptoms, if any, occurred. Be sure to **drink
   enough water** — dehydration can cause headaches, dizziness,
   and light-headedness.

4. **At the end of the three-day period, make an assessment.** Did
   you feel better, worse, or the same? If you felt better, you are on
   the right track and can move ahead with the diet, adding one
   new food every three days, rotating between protein, starch/
   grain, vegetable, and fruit. By the end of the first week you'll get
   the hang of it.

5. **If you felt worse or the same, you may be allergic or sensitive
   to one of these four or five foods.** Do not substitute a legume,
   nut, egg, shellfish (including shrimp), or citrus fruit for any of
   your choices, as all are likely to produce allergic reactions. These
   foods should only be tried toward the end of your allergy elimination diet, when you already have a wide variety of safe foods
   to eat.

6. **When you're ready to add new foods, consider choosing from
   the suggestions below:**
   - *Some good vegetable choices include:* parsnips, carrots, celery,
     zucchini, celery root, lettuce, jicama, cauliflower, and broccoli.
     Asparagus isn't a good choice, as it is a diuretic and is very likely
     to increase urinary frequency. If you are not bothered by vegeta-
     bles high in oxalates, then spinach and kale are excellent choices.
   - *Good fruit choices include:* apples, pears, peaches, mangoes,
     papaya, blueberries, and sour cherries. Melon, pineapple, and
     citrus are not good choices for beginning the allergy elimination
     diet. However, you can use watermelon for its diuretic proper-
     ties if you suffer from abdominal bloating or water retention —
     just make sure you have bathroom access.
   - *Almonds and Brazil nuts are good choices for nuts, if you do not
     have an allergy to tree nuts:* Almond milk, hazelnut milk, or
     hemp milk may be a good substitute for dairy. Peanuts, which
     are highly allergenic, are *not* a good choice, and pistachios and
     cashews can also trigger allergic reactions. Walnuts can be

added fairly early on. When using nuts, be careful to inspect them carefully; avoid dark, discolored nuts, which may be rancid or contain mold. Rancid nuts, and oils made from them, also have an "off" odor and taste and should be avoided.

- *Seasonings:* Stick to herbs, preferably fresh, for at least a few weeks. It will make it easier to tell exactly which foods you are reacting to. For example, if you are testing chicken, and you add forty cloves of garlic to it, you aren't just testing the chicken, are you? Many people are quite sensitive to garlic and onions. A few people even react to basil or cilantro. Sea salt is a wonderful complex seasoning, much preferable to table salt, and it contains a wider array of naturally occurring minerals.

Hopefully, by the end of the first month you will become aware of which "groups" of foods you react to and will still have plenty of variety in your diet. These "reactive" foods may be nightshades (peppers, eggplant, tomatoes, potatoes), citrus fruits, foods that contain vasoactive amines, like dark red-skinned fruits, red wine, chocolate, aged foods, etc., or they may all be grains. Perhaps you can't tolerate any grains at this point, until your gut heals. A pattern will develop — trust me on this. You may have a huge number of food sensitivities, but keep in mind that this will not always be the case. As your gut heals in the absence of gluten and/or casein, you will eventually lose your sensitivity to a number of foods.

The elimination diet process takes a deep commitment, planning, and organization, but it can yield some impressive results as you methodically track down every irritant, allergy, and food sensitivity. This approach may be a necessity for those suffering from multiple food sensitivities that could be affecting their bladder symptoms.

To make things easier, I've included a modified allergy elimination diet plan below.

An Easy Alternative: A Modified Elimination Diet

This is the fastest, most efficient way to eliminate possible bladder irritants from your diet. Make a sincere effort to follow a modified elimination diet for two to three weeks. Rather than starting from scratch, start by eliminating from your diet all sources of the top

eight allergens: milk, eggs, peanuts, tree nuts (almonds, walnuts, pecans, etc.), wheat, soy, fish, and shellfish.

In addition, it is a good idea to also exclude corn, a common allergen, and cane sugar, a common bladder irritant. For those crying
out loud, "What's left to eat?" the answer is the following:

- every *fruit* on the planet, except those you know irritate your
  bladder, such as citrus fruits and cranberries
- every *vegetable* on the planet, except perhaps some nightshade
  vegetables, or those high in oxalates, such as spinach, as well as a
  multitude of salad greens
- many forms of *protein*, such as chicken, turkey, beef, lamb, buf-
  falo, wild game, and legumes
- wholesome nutritious *grains* like quinoa, wild rice, brown rice,
  and oats (unless you are sensitive or know you are gluten-intolerant and aren't sure you should eat oats)

That covers a whole lot of culinary ground, and you can supplement with well-tolerated seasonings, healthy oils, and fresh herbs.

After eliminating the top allergens for a few weeks, begin introducing foods from the suggestions above one item at a time, every three days. This modified diet isn't considered a strict elimination diet, but it should prove very useful for many people to try for
a short period. *Always check with your health practitioner first before
attempting to follow an elimination diet. This is especially important
if you are a diabetic or suffer from hypoglycemia, anemia, or another
metabolic disorder.*

It is important to plan and shop ahead to successfully complete
an elimination diet. Being hungry and irritable—feeling deprived—
may lead you to give up the diet before you are able to obtain the answers you are looking for.

What You Can Do Now

Who better than you to figure out what's bugging your bladder? A
good way to take responsibility for your own health is to begin keeping a diet journal. It isn't concerned with calories, so you don't need

to include amounts, just the foods themselves, and don't forget beverages too. Make up your own diet plans and take good notes on your reactions. The profound effect of diet and exercise on health and well-being cannot be overestimated. You may be surprised by the results!

By following this modified elimination diet plan, you may realize that, like many people with IC, you are very sensitive to gluten and need to avoid eating gluten-containing foods entirely. Or, you may discover that you are sensitive to histamines or oxalates or nightshades. Take advantage of the diet information presented in this chapter and in the Resources section at the conclusion of the book. There are also numerous web-based resources presenting a variety of specialty diets. Just keep in mind that your individual dietary needs and food sensitivities may be very particular. We're all unique, and we need to learn to eat as consciously as possible for our own health. Admittedly, individual needs can increase the complexity of planning and preparing meals for a family, but taking the extra time to really think about food in this way can repay our efforts with fewer trips to the doctor, less time off from work, and greatly improved health.

14

You *Can* Get Well

When my children were very young and suffering a childhood illness, my father-in-law used to calm my fears by telling me that there is a difference between a really sick child and a healthy child who is simply ill. There is a similar continuum of illness in adults. For many years, when my IC symptoms were not so bad, I considered myself a healthy, vibrant person who happened to have an illness that flared up now and then. I had young children to raise, a home to remodel, a challenging career as a hospital nurse, and a variety of interests I wished to pursue. Keeping the attitude that I was not "chronically ill" was very important to my sense of self. And I have to believe that maintaining this attitude helped to boost my outlook on life, helped me deal with the frustration and pain of IC, and for many years helped me avoid sustained periods of depression. In contrast, at the height of my illness, I began to lose the sense of myself as a healthy person who simply had an illness. This transition seems to be common in chronically ill people, but believe me when I say that such an attitude can lead to a very dark place, one that is best avoided.

Keep a Healthy Outlook

Many people are unaware that when a deficiency in neurotransmitters results in depression, the imbalance can trigger physical symptoms, too, so it is really important to your recovery to do what you can to bolster your spirits. Maintaining positivity means having faith in your ability to get well. Surround yourself with others who provide assurance that you *will* get through any temporary setbacks and that you *will* recover. As much as possible, keep in mind the following principle as you approach your recovery from IC and other sources of chronic pelvic pain (CPP):

> *Never give up the belief that you can recover. Your recovery may be partial or it may be complete, but no matter how ill you have been, you have within you the power to heal and to move toward recovery. In holding to this principle, it is sometimes necessary to walk away from a medical practitioner who hints, or states outright, that you are not going to get any better.*

The following is Bob's story, just one of many that make this point:

CASE STUDY: *Bob*

I'm a male IC patient and have had chronic symptoms for the past six years. One urologist prescribed the usual antibiotics for over a year, even without evidence of infection. When that was unsuccessful, my urologist jumped to the conclusion that the problem was with my prostate, even though it checked out to be normal. At that point, I changed to a new urologist and asked to be tested for IC, since my sister has suffered from the condition for many years. Finally, a bladder biopsy was performed, confirming IC. At my doctor's recommendation I went on Elmiron for several years before deciding it was causing more problems than it was helping. I ordered a book on the suggested IC diet from the IC network (see Resources), but after eliminating all of the common bladder irritants from my diet I was still not seeing any positive results. By this time, I was undergoing hydrodistentions every three months, and I had developed painful Hunner's ulcers on my bladder wall. I changed urologists once again, and my new urologist said my only alternative was to have my bladder removed!

I went searching for another doctor and began investigating any other sources of food that could be causing irritation. I found a great doctor, and I also discovered a website in Australia that stated that

(cont'd.)

avoiding all dairy products would eliminate 75 percent of the pain and other problems associated with IC. I have now gone one year without eating any dairy products—that means no ice cream, butter, cream, or baked goods containing milk products. I use Rice Dream as a milk substitute. The pain from IC has decreased with each month while I have been on this dairy-restricted diet.

I'm now going five months between hydrodistentions. My last hydrodistention was very positive, and the doctor doesn't expect me back for six months. I also have a lot of friends and family praying for me. I am very thankful for finding that website from Australia, which allowed me to get on the path to recovery.

The frightening thing about this story is that if Bob had followed his doctor's advice to have his bladder removed, he would have undergone a fairly risky surgery with a possibility of postoperative infection, and the loss of his bladder would have been permanent. There's no going back from bladder-removal surgery! Another important thing for someone in Bob's position to consider is that for many patients, this type of major surgery is not a permanent cure for pain, inflammation, and other IC symptoms. Some patients continue to experience pelvic pain even after the bladder is removed. This is actually not surprising when you consider factors such as neurogenic inflammation, hyperexcitability of the pelvic nerves, and the generalized inflammation that may be an immune-driven response to food allergies. While Bob's story isn't typical, it shows that even a severe case of IC can improve and that making positive changes to your overall health is important—especially before resorting to a drastic measure such as bladder-removal surgery.

Ask for the Kind of Help You Need

Most of us have been brought up with the Western-medicine model. Sadly, modern medicine seems to pay too little attention to efficient and accurate diagnosis, based on physical assessment and listening to the patient (one of the lost arts of medicine), and often turns too quickly to pharmaceutical intervention. The problem with this approach is that no "miracle pill" exists for many chronic diseases, including IC. Elmiron (discussed in Chapter 3) was once held in such high hopes, but it is not as promising as first thought. If you've exhausted the conventional advice of allopathic physicians, where do you turn? A second important principle to keep in mind is the following:

> *IC and chronic pelvic pain affect your whole self, so it is important to find a way to treat your whole self. If you're very fortunate, you can do this with a single wise practitioner, or you may need to enlist the help of a competent and caring health-care team.*

A doctor who looks in your bladder and says, "Yes, you have IC," and sends you home with a prescription for Elmiron (and maybe one for the antihistamine hydroxyzine) is not looking at your whole self, and he or she is not going to be able to help you fully recover from IC. Can you ever stop taking the Elmiron? If not, then you aren't recovered. You're just on medication, a very expensive medication that takes a long time to work, has significant side effects, and isn't of great benefit to a large number of IC patients. If your doctor hasn't asked you about any other area of your life—what responsibilities you have, what stresses you're experiencing, and what other health conditions you suffer from, no matter how minor—then your doctor can't possibly be seeing the big picture of your overall health, your IC, or any other CPP.

If any of the medical doctors I'd been to had really taken time to investigate my condition holistically, they'd have discovered that I had multiple food sensitivities and allergies, chronic sinus problems, chronic migraines, a history of ongoing antibiotic use prior to the onset of my IC, which I suspect led to my "leaky gut," which, in turn, led to all those food sensitivities. They would have seen a pattern of immune system hyperreactivity, which can be a precursor to autoimmune disorders and other types of chronic disease. One physician prescribed nearly three months of antibiotics for repeat strep infections, including scarlet fever. Yes, I was very ill and antibiotics were necessary. However, if he had also worked with me to rebuild my immunity, might I have avoided going on to become chronically ill? Perhaps. But I know now that I would have been much better off with a healthy gut, which is where the majority of our immune system exerts its protective effects. Rebuilding a healthy gut after destruction of the intestinal flora takes time and effort. Eating some yogurt for breakfast occasionally is a good idea, but doing so is not nearly enough.

Asking for the kind of help you need means being resourceful, being hopeful, being open-minded, and being a little bit of a detective. It means asking for help from others you know who have battled chronic illness. Word of mouth is a great way to obtain a recommendation for a new health practitioner. Trust your friends' recommendations, but at the same time, realize that not every doctor-to-patient relationship is a perfect match. You do not have to love the doctor your neighbor is wild about.

True healers are very special people, and it doesn't necessarily matter what initials they have after their name. Still, you must maintain some degree of skepticism and common sense in order to avoid those who may try to take advantage of you. Do not order expensive supplements or other untried products online. *Never* allow yourself to feel vulnerable in a situation that makes you uncomfortable, either in the way you are treated by any member of the staff, or by the lack of cleanliness or order in a medical office. Trust your instincts, and act on them.

Below is a success story from someone who found help by continually searching for answers. Suzy didn't give up, and her hard work paid off!

CASE STUDY: *Suzy*

Halleluja! After ten years of debilitating symptoms—stomach pain, chronic constipation, cystitis that kept me up all night, and kidney inflammation and pain—the explanation I found on your website regarding food sensitivities (especially gluten) and the bladder was the first one that made sense. I have been to dozens of doctors, conventional and otherwise, have been on Biltricide, Diflucan, and other antiparasitic and antifungal medications, but every time I stopped the anti-candida diet that I've been following on and off for the last five years I'd be back to square one. (Note: The anti-candida diet strictly limits grains and sugars.) Surely this is enough time to have starved a fungus! I have acupuncture once a week to help the pain in my legs and lower back, and the most painful meridians are always bladder, kidneys, and stomach. I finally began to work out that my problems are diet related, not necessarily candida-related, and that I'm reacting to wheat, dairy, and sugars. I'm also sensitive to some animal proteins. Basically, I do best following a mostly vegetarian diet, and I can tolerate legumes and some grains, but not wheat, dairy, or red meat. I have been advised by many practitioners to follow the blood-type diet, and this is essentially what I do best with, even though I had previously been skeptical. Now that I realize I'm sensitive to specific groups of foods that were not traditionally eaten by my blood type, I have a better understanding of my body's dietary needs. Thank you for making clear to me the connection between food sensitivities and the bladder.

Appeal to a Higher Power

[*Ask for help from a higher power, whether you call it fate, the Universe, God, or your personal spirit guide(s).*]

There's another source of help you can consult at any time, and that's the Universe. Remember the old saying "Be careful what you wish for, because you just might get it?" There is a power in hope and belief. Norman Vincent Peale called it the power of positive thinking. Simply ask for what you need — precisely and without hesitation. Focus on true needs rather than wants. You may want a new dress, but what you need is a truly skilled health practitioner who understands you, listens to you, and has the insights to be able to help you in your recovery. So go ahead and ask for that person to come into your life.

If you're spiritually inclined, ask your priest or minister to pray for you, and ask for help by praying yourself. Many religious traditions set aside special services for healing, and these rituals can have powerful healing effects. Ask your friends and family members to pray for you, as Bob, in the earlier story, has done.

Sometimes the answer is just around the corner. Maybe consciously asking for what we need makes us more aware so that we recognize what we're looking for when we see it. Or maybe there's more to it. I'll let you be the judge.

Experience Healing Day by Day

I don't claim that recovering from chronic pelvic pain is easy, or that it is a straightforward, one-size-fits-all process. Rather, I have tried throughout this book to make the point that you must keep searching for your particular answer, keep "turning over stones." However, I can make it a little easier by outlining a "day in the life" of someone following the principles in this book. It is all very doable and within your control. *You* must be the one to guide your own healing process, using the knowledge you've now gained about your illness and the ways in which diet, stress, hormones, occult infections, and many other factors affect your health. Let's take a look at how you can begin taking the first steps to wellness.

Today you may be waking up after a restless night, with many trips to the bathroom and pain that has prevented you from falling back to sleep easily. Lie in bed for a few minutes and take several deep breaths, inhaling through your nose and exhaling through your mouth, energizing and awakening your body, while at the same time calming your nervous system. Move slowly when getting up, allowing yourself a gentle start to the day. Stretch tall, arms overhead, bending your spine in the four directions while gently stretching your lower abdomen. Say to yourself, "I'm going to get well, beginning today. It may take a sustained effort, but my health is worth it, I'm worth it, and I deserve to be well!" Let this be your daily positive affirmation.

Practice sitting in a squatting position a few times to gently stretch out those pelvic floor muscles, which may have been clenching tight all night long. One easy way to do this is to grab the morning newspaper or a light book and head to your nearest heat register for a warm and cozy few minutes, while you continue to do some breathing exercises, focusing on relaxing those muscles. You are priming them for the day, telling them what you want them to do, which is to relax and stay relaxed. Instead of tensing your pelvic floor, take this moment to affirm that you will handle stress in other ways, by writing it down, verbally expressing it in an appropriate fashion, or finding another healthy solution.

Now it is time to visit the bathroom and use some pH paper to test your early morning urine. If it is below 6.2, add a pinch of baking soda (¼ teaspoon or less) to a big glass of room-temperature water to help alkalize your urine.

While you are brushing your teeth, think of ways to decrease stress. If listening to the morning news of car crashes, child molestation, murder, war casualties, and other atrocities doesn't brighten your day (and why would it?), then turn off the radio and put on some music instead. My husband prefers classical, while I prefer jazz and ethnic music. In warm weather, open the windows and listen to morning birdsong—the most beautiful music on earth. I've recently stopped listening to the morning news in the car on my way to work, and I now listen to a delightful CD of sounds of nature. I find it very calming.

Make a light alkaline breakfast. Your body is most acidic in the early morning hours and upon rising. Enjoy a tall glass of almond milk, a salad of fresh fruit and nuts, a plate of sliced jicama, or, one of my favorites, a carrot-jicama-apple salad. Coconut yogurt is a soothing alternative to soy or dairy, and combining it with fruit into a smoothie with a little flaxseed meal or flaxseed oil is delicious. Avoid beginning your day with inflammatory foods like eggs, high-sodium breakfast meats, or high-glycemic sweetened baked goods. Why get started on the wrong track?

Make time in your busy schedule to do some simple stretches or yoga poses, maintaining your calm demeanor. Then, take a big step. Make an appointment with a naturopath or other practitioner who can test you for food sensitivities. Get started on your own individualized healing path right away. Whether it is gluten, soy, eggs, or sugar, finding out what's bugging your bladder is one of the most important keys to your recovery.

During your morning break time, avoid caffeine and sugary, gluten-filled snacks—fuel for the fires in your bladder—and stick to the water cooler instead. You could also choose to brew a soothing cup of herbal tea. While you're standing there, or whenever you think of it throughout the day, check in with your pelvic floor. Are you holding tension there, clenching the muscles and squeezing your poor bladder? Stop! Take a deep breath. Consciously feel the elevator of your pelvic floor drop a few levels. Do a few minutes of deep breathing. Anxiety naturally triggers us to tense our pelvic floor. It happens to everyone. For those with IC and pelvic floor dysfunction, it is a repetitive pattern that leads to increased pelvic pain. Tensing the pelvic floor muscles can tend to go along with clenching the jaw and grinding the teeth. These are all responses to stress and anxiety, so watch out for these telltale signs, too.

At lunch time, eat a big green salad with a little olive oil and a pinch of sea salt. Vegetables can add flavors of their own. You don't need vinegar, which may only irritate your bladder. You can purchase several varieties of vinegar-free salad dressing, or you can make your own using apple juice, apple cider, or mild-tasting pear juice (no sugar added!) in place of vinegar. Mix a few teaspoons of good-quality mayonnaise with a few drops of sesame oil and a tablespoon of olive oil or canola oil; thin the mixture with some apple or pear juice. Toss in a few poppy seeds, and you will have a delicious vinegar-free poppy-seed dressing. If you can tolerate a squeeze of lemon juice, or a dash of wheat-free tamari soy sauce, try these for variety. These flavors combine well with oil and salt to make a quick dressing. Include some fresh organic turkey in your salad if you need protein. It is less likely than many other animal proteins to cause food allergies and sensitivities (but you still need to be tested). A handful of almonds or walnuts is another protein option. Drink more water after lunch. See how eating such a healthful, alkaline meal makes you feel during the afternoon.

Throughout your workday, be aware of how long you are sitting in one position, and be aware of your posture, in general. Avoid putting prolonged pressure on the pelvic floor muscles. Get up often and stretch, and practice mini-shifts in position, moving slightly in one direction or another to take pressure off a given area. Ask about seating alternatives. Maybe you can bring in an exercise ball, a kneel-on chair, or a memory-foam pillow to put on your desk chair.

As much as possible, avoid stressful traffic on the ride home. Take the scenic route, if possible. Make sure you empty your bladder before getting into the car for a long commute. If you have time on your way home, stop and pick up some healing herbs for the bladder. Linden is a great all-around choice, but there are many other helpful, soothing herbs for the bladder, including ordinary chamomile (more information on herbs is located in Appendix B).

Eat a healthful dinner, following the 80/20 principle of the anti-inflammatory diet. Protein is important, but most animal protein is acid-producing, so it needs to be balanced by a larger portion of alkaline plant foods.

After dinner, take a fairly long, fairly brisk walk. Walk off the frustrations of the day, breathe fresh air, and spend time in nature with your children, your sweetheart, a good friend, or a family pet. Nurture yourself with loving relationships and time spent simply enjoying life.

Drink ample water throughout the day, but begin to wind down by dinnertime. After dinner, make a cup of mild linden-flower tea or chamomile tea and sip it slowly. Stop drinking liquids at least an hour or two before bedtime so that you have time to void.

Unless you have sodium-associated high blood pressure, drink a small glass of water with baking soda in it before bedtime. (If you are fairly alkaline, drinking water with baking soda isn't necessary, and you don't need the extra sodium.) If sleep is a real problem for you, as it is for so many, follow some of the sleep hygiene suggestions given in the book. These include taking a warm bath with Epsom salts before bedtime, and possibly taking some sleep supplements such as 5-HTP, melatonin, or valerian. If you suffer from bladder spasms, consider using one of the antispasmodic herbs mentioned earlier, such as ashwagandha or skullcap, but first educate yourself in their use by reading all about them in Appendix B, a comprehensive guide to herbs for the bladder.

As you lie down to sleep, try one of the relaxation exercises I've suggested, such as relaxing from the toes up. Pay special attention to how your pelvic floor muscles feel and spend a few minutes doing deep abdominal breathing to work on normalizing the muscle response of your pelvic floor. This can do wonders to prevent the spasms that wake you at night with a sudden urge to void.

Sleep well, and wake up feeling a bit more rested and a bit more hopeful. Repeat.

These simple changes in your daily routine will begin to turn things around for you. If you continue this routine, methodically track down your food sensitivities, work toward hormonal balance, and eliminate the possibility of occult infections, Lyme disease, and candida overgrowth, you will begin to heal not only your bladder, but perhaps other health problems as well, including fatigue, achy joints, headaches, and mood swings. It takes work and commitment, but let the work of getting well replace the difficulty of living with chronic illness.

I always tell my children that "anything worth having is worth working for." It is a principle I live by, and having good health is no exception. We've all heard the saying, "If you have your health, you have everything." In so many ways it is true. I've had good health and I've had terrible health. Good health is so much better. It is truly worth everything.

Measure Success by Your Own Standards

What are your standards for living a healthy, active life? Only you can answer that question. For me, it was being able to return to my career and to the dynamic, outdoor lifestyle I loved. It was also very important for me to be a more active and involved parent of two sons, and a better partner to my spouse. In 1995 I knew I had IC, and in 1996 I received my diagnosis. By 2002 my IC was so bad that it became increasingly difficult to keep working. However, I have now fully recovered, and I have written this book to help others reach the same success.

I have been an avid backpacker since 1978, when I moved from Pennsylvania to the mountains of Colorado to attend college. My husband and I have logged hundreds of miles toting backpacks holding everything from botanical guides and binoculars to small children and diapers. Our two sons once held a mutiny in the mountains of New Mexico, stating that our next vacation would be in a fancy hotel with a swimming pool (it never happened!). Finally, mostly because of my IC, I said I couldn't do it anymore. The pressure of my pack's waistband had grown so uncomfortable that I had been adjusting the straps to carry most of the weight on my shoulders. This led to pressure on the nerves there, which ultimately caused problems too difficult to ignore. Furthermore, I could no longer sit comfortably on a bike seat despite having a nifty mountain bike that I loved. I felt like I'd given up a significant part of myself. My husband, who proposed to me with a brand-new bicycle rather than an engagement ring, felt like he'd lost his recreation partner. Things looked bleak — for both of us and for our marriage. I had quite a few fears for my future.

I began taking all the steps discussed throughout this book. It wasn't always easy or straightforward, but I didn't have a book like this to follow. I discovered many sources discussing individual aspects of healing (which I mention in the Acknowledgments and Resources). The key was figuring out what my body needed and designing my own plan for healing. (Actually, I designed many plans. No one achieves perfect success on the first try.)

In May 2008 I backpacked with my husband through Cedar Mesa in southeastern Utah for our twentieth anniversary. My ability to do so without discomfort meant a lot to both of us. For the past three summers I've enjoyed riding my mountain bike to the farmer's market in a nearby town. Two years ago I took up running again to chase away the winter blues and to prevent my usual seasonal ten-pound weight gain. And I continue to be able to swim all the way across the cold, cold lake in northwestern Montana where we vacation each summer. Rather than facing a future as an older adult who isn't capable of living the life she's dreamed of, I'm facing my fifties with the hope that if I keep to the path I'm on, the outlook is bright. I wish the same for you.

Final Words

Please contact me through my publisher, Hunter House, and let me know how you are doing. I know many of you face special challenges, but *everyone* is capable of some degree of healing, and many, many people will be able to recover from chronic illness with a holistic approach such as the one presented in this book. This plan worked for me, and it will work for you, too. It is based on sound science, not solely on my own personal idiosyncrasies. I've offered a broadly holistic approach, with many possible options to help you to design your own specific plan for healing. A journey begins with a single step, so take that step. You deserve to live a healthy life, free of chronic pain.

Getting Started on a Gluten-Free Diet

I strongly recommend following a strict gluten-free diet if you suffer from IC or chronic prostatitis. The information in this Appendix is reprinted from my book *Gluten-Free Portland — A Resource Guide.* Please see this book for helpful meal-planning tips and menu suggestions. It is available through my website www.glutenfreechoice.com.

Foods That Contain Gluten — To Be Avoided on a Gluten-Free Diet

In advising clients how to live a gluten-free lifestyle, I tend to focus on the positives, like what we *can* eat. Of course, it is also critical to know which specific foods to avoid, rather than just the broad categories of wheat, rye, barley, etc. I've included a list of foods to avoid, hidden sources of gluten, and even information on medications. Readers interested in learning more about gluten intolerance and about following a gluten-free diet can access further information on my website, www.thebetterbladder bookinfo.com.

Breads and Starches to Avoid
- bread crumbs (unless made from gluten-free bread)
- any bread made from wheat, barley, rye, oats (unless certified gluten-free), or "multi-grain"(including spelt)
- cereals including muesli, oatmeal, farina, cream of wheat, dry cereals that contain wheat, barley, rye, or oats, including most popular brands
- any cereal or other food that contains "malt," "malt extract," or "malt flavoring"
- couscous and whole-wheat couscous
- crackers and trail mixes, bridge mixes that contain crackers, bread rounds, or pita chips, unless specifically labeled gluten-free

- packaged rice and pasta mixes (e.g., Rice-a-Roni, ramen noodles, Hamburger Helper)
- pretzels (unless labeled gluten-free)
- whole-wheat or flour tortillas
- breads, salads, or soups that contain wheat, barley, bulgur (wheat) — e.g., tabouli salad
- all flours that contain wheat, barley, rye, or oats, including white flour, cake flour, unbleached flour, bread flour, self-rising flour, graham flour, semolina flour, pastry flour
- durum flour, gluten flour, gluten, wheat gluten, vital gluten, barley flour, light or dark rye flour, oat flour, spelt flour, oat bran, wheat germ, wheat bran, triticale, wheat starch, kamut (gluten-free oats can now be purchased — see "All about Grains" on page 251)
- any noodle or pasta of any size or shape that isn't labeled gluten-free. Quinoa, corn, Jerusalem artichoke, buckwheat, and brown rice pastas are all possibilities that are usually safe, but be sure to check the labeling for any additives or binders that may contain gluten. *Pay special attention to rice blends that may contain wheat berries.*

Dairy Foods and Beverages to Avoid

- chocolate drinks, hot cocoa mix, chocolate milk
- malted milk drinks and shakes, mixes like instant breakfast and protein drinks
- flavored yogurt drinks and kefir (may contain gluten)
- Post-um and other grain-based coffee substitutes
- teas like Roastaroma made from roasted barley, any tea containing roasted barley or barley malt or malt flavoring
- teas from tea bags that have crimped edges glued together with wheat starch; safest bets are tea bags sewn together, or folded and stapled together
- beer, ale, and malt liquor contain gluten — there are now gluten-free beers on the market
- blue (Bleu) cheese — the lines of mold may be produced using wheat flour as a growth medium — check with manufacturer
- caramel-colored soft drinks like colas and root beer, especially if made outside the United States — there are some high-end specialty brands of root beer that are labeled gluten-free, including Virgil's

Fruits and Vegetables to Avoid

- baby foods with starch or pasta added
- baby cereals, except for rice
- breaded vegetables and frozen breaded vegetables
- creamed soups or creamed vegetables, like pearl onions
- spreads with thickeners (may contain gluten)
- any fruit pie, pastry, or cobbler with a crust, crumb topping, or filling thickener
- French fries, unless made at home or in a dedicated fryer. Even packaged French fries, hash browns, and home fries sometimes contain wheat starch to keep them from sticking together
- flavored potato chips and other kinds of chips, like Sun Chips

Protein Sources to Avoid

- breaded meat, fish, chicken, turkey, and soy products, like Morning Star Farms Chix Patties
- canned pork and beans (except Bush's or other gluten-free brands)
- casseroles made with pasta, dumplings, biscuit topping, Bisquik, or gravy (usually thickened with flour)
- chicken, turkey, hot dogs, veggie hot dogs, or other deli processed meat products like Yves Deli Slices—usually made with wheat gluten or gluten additives (the additives are in the broth used in manufacture or packaging for moistness)
- imitation bacon, imitation seafood ("sea-legs" or "krab"), imitation ham, processed meats
- meat dishes or casseroles in which bread crumbs or gravies have been used, such as meatloaf, Swiss steak, meatballs, and salmon patties, unless you make them yourself
- TVP (texturized vegetable protein) and seitan (made from wheat gluten)
- Any "veggie burger" not explicitly labeled gluten-free

Desserts to Avoid

- all cookies, pastries, cakes, pies, cobblers, and bars made with any type of flour that isn't expressly labeled gluten-free or that you did not grind yourself from a gluten-free grain; this includes spelt, which is often marketed as "wheat-free," as spelt contains gluten.

- any dessert whose filling may have been thickened with flour, or non-specified starch, or modified food starch not made from a gluten-free grain
- ice cream and ice-cream cones, unless homemade or carefully labeled; sorbet is a better alternative, but check the ingredients anyway
- licorice, jellybeans, and other gummy candies, unless identified as gluten-free
- chocolate bars — can often contain gluten and dairy, but it is now possible to buy gluten-free chocolate

Condiments, Seasonings, and Additives (Hidden Sources) to Avoid

- dried soup mixes, especially those made with noodles
- most canned soups and dry soup mixes, bouillon mixes and soup bases made with yeast or vegetable protein
- salad dressings that contain malt vinegar or vinegar distilled from grain — read the label
- chip dips other than salsa or homemade guacamole or hummus
- gravies and sauces, cream sauces, béchamel sauce
- seasoning packets and mixes — make your own or buy simple herbal blends
- chili sauce, steak sauce, and soy sauce (unless labeled gluten-free or wheat-free)
- rice syrup or brown rice syrup, if not labeled gluten-free (sometimes contains barley malt)
- some pickled foods
- many prepared mustards (read labels carefully)
- flavorings and colorings can contain gluten, especially caramel flavoring and caramel coloring, and malt flavoring or malt extract (unless identified) — annatto (orange) and beet juice (red/purple) colorings are okay
- malt vinegar; most other vinegars do not contain gluten
- some spice blends, such as curry powder, lemon pepper, etc., may contain starches as fillers (may contain gluten) — you can buy pure spices and mix your own
- nondairy creamers; check ingredient lists — some newer products are soy or coconut milk based and are gluten-free

- emulsifiers, stabilizers, and binders, unless clearly identified as gluten-free
- vegetable gums, thickeners, or starches, unless identified as gluten-free
- hydrolyzed vegetable protein (HVP), texturized vegetable protein (TVP), and hydrolyzed plant protein (HPP)
- dextrin, maltodextrin (usually derived from corn in the United States, but not elsewhere — check with the manufacturer for specs; okay if derived from corn)
- modified food starch — may be derived from wheat or from nongluten grains — check with manufacturer
- monoglycerides and diglycerides — safe if made in the United States; may contain gluten if made with other processes elsewhere
- anticaking agents and dispersing agents — unless identified as gluten-free
- wheat-germ oil or vitamin-E oil
- chewing gum may or may not contain gluten, so reading labels is crucial. Trident and Wrigley have gluten-free options. Check manufacturer website FAQs

Supplements and Pharmaceuticals to Avoid

Gluten in supplements, pharmaceutical medications, and over-the-counter drugs comes primarily from fillers and binders. Any product that contains the word "starch" as an inactive ingredient may be suspect. Common ingredients that may contain gluten also include "dextrins," "maltodextrin," and "pregelatinized starch." For more information, read package inserts carefully, and see the following websites:

www.glutenfreedrugs.com
www.stokesrx.com
www.practicalgastro.com

To obtain accurate information on whether your prescription or over-the-counter medications contain gluten, speak with your pharmacist.

All About Grains

Regular baking flour (white flour) is always made from wheat. Spelt is a form of wheat, kamut is a form of wheat, couscous is wheat (pasta), and semolina is wheat, no matter how trendy they are or how highly recommended they come. Spelt, in particular, has become the darling of the alternative food industry, and many foods marked "wheat-free" are in fact made from spelt, which is not gluten-free. While spelt holds promise as an "ancient grain" that is both lower in gluten and easier to digest, and may someday form the basis of a truly gluten-free wheat that is safe for gluten-intolerant people, we aren't there yet—all people with celiac disease or gluten-intolerance should avoid eating spelt.

While oats do not contain the same form of gluten that wheat contains, they contain a similar protein called avenin, which the body's immune system may mistake for gluten, causing sensitivity in some individuals. Oats, like many grains, can also be contaminated with wheat or other gluten-containing grains, by being grown in fields where wheat was previously grown, or by being milled or processed on shared equipment. This is unfortunate because oats are both nutritious and delicious, and oat flour is a wonderful and economical 1:1 substitute for wheat flour. Recently, it has become possible to buy oats that are not contaminated with gluten, though they are more expensive. If you try certified gluten-free oats after being gluten-free for a while, do so cautiously and listen to your body. Look for gluten-free oats online, at Bob's Red Mill, or at higher-end health-food stores.

There are a lot of "alternative" baked good products on the market, many of them local, nutritious, and delicious, but they may not be gluten-free. Information on "Grains to Avoid" is repeated below. When choosing alternative grains or baked goods, remember the following:

Grains to Avoid

- *Barley* isn't gluten-free.
- *Faro (or farro)* isn't gluten-free.
- *Kamut* isn't gluten-free—it is a form of wheat and contains gluten.
- *Oats* do not necessarily mean gluten-free (see above). There are now three brands of gluten-free oats advertised: Gifts of Nature certified gluten-free oats, Lara's Gluten-Free rolled oats from Cream Hill Estates, and Glutenfreeoats.com.
- *Rye* isn't gluten-free.
- *Semolina* isn't gluten-free—it is a form of wheat and contains gluten.
- *Spelt* isn't gluten-free—it is a form of wheat and contains gluten, although a smaller percentage than regular wheat.
- *Wheat-free* does not necessarily mean gluten-free, as some wheat-free items can contain other forms of gluten such as barley malt.

Safe Gluten-Free Grains and Flours

- *almond flour*
- *amaranth*: tiny seeds — also available as a flour
- *bean flours*: garbanzo, red bean, white bean, etc.
- *coconut flour*
- *corn*: corn meal, grits, corn masa
- *hazelnut flour*
- *millet*: milled whole grains, or ground into flour
- *montina* (expensive, but nice if you can find it)
- *potato starch*
- *quinoa*: whole grains, traditional brown or Inca Red, flaked (like rolled oats), or flour
- *rice*: brown, white, basmati, jasmine, wild, purple, black, and red
- *sorghum*: brown or white, it makes a good additive to gluten-free flour mixes
- *tapioca flour/tapioca starch*: finely ground tapioca, also tapioca pearls (tiny pellets of dried processed tapioca)
- *teff*: the traditional grain of northern Africa — also available as a flour

The Nutritional Content of Grains

Whole grains in general are good sources of carbohydrates and minerals such as magnesium and selenium, but one of their most important nutritional benefits is the fiber they bring to our diets. Whole grains such as wheat, brown rice, and oats include both soluble and insoluble fiber. Soluble fiber is easy to remember — it is water soluble, and as such can be assimilated into the body, where it plays an important role in blood sugar regulation and cholesterol balance. Soluble fiber also helps provide a sense of fullness or satiety. Insoluble fiber is — you guessed it — insoluble in water, and instead of being assimilated into the body it passes through the digestive tract and is eliminated. That does not mean insoluble fiber has a less important nutritional role to play; rather, insoluble fiber is very important in keeping our digestive and elimination systems regular. In doing so, fiber helps aid the transit of toxic substances out of the body. This process, when operating optimally, helps to reduce the incidence of colon and rectal cancers.

In eliminating gluten grains from your diet, have you wondered what you are missing nutritionally? Are you able to get adequate replacements for the nutrients in wheat, barley, rye, and oats from the other nutritional components of your diet? The answer is a qualified "Yes." For tens of thousands of years, entire cultures have thrived without growing or consuming any of the gluten grains. We also know, from looking at what nutrients gluten grains provide, that there are more than adequate sources of these nutrients in alternative grains and from vegetable sources. Fiber is something we do need to be aware of, though. Studies have shown that standard gluten-free diets are low in fiber, especially when baking with the "white" alternative products like white or sweet rice flour, tapioca starch, and potato starch, which provide little nutrition and almost no fiber. We can remedy this by eating alternative grains in whole, unprocessed states, and by including nuts, seeds, and other sources of fiber such as dried fruit, ground flax seed, and legumes in our diets.

When making your flour blends, coming up with new recipes, and altering traditional wheat-flour recipes, try to include alternative grain products (and sometimes nut flours) that contain substantial amounts of fiber, protein, calcium, and iron, all nutrients found in whole grains, but in much smaller amounts in highly processed grains. Quinoa, sorghum, teff, amaranth, brown rice, and millet flour are all nutritious grains to cook and bake with.

Setting Up Your Gluten-Free Kitchen

Life would be easier if everyone in your family followed the same diet, but this usually isn't the case. Fortunately, gluten intolerance rarely causes the kinds of immediately life-threatening allergic reactions we sometimes read about. However, the amount of gluten that can trigger symptoms is still very tiny—the size of a sesame seed! Some people are even more sensitive, and they have to be extremely careful to avoid even being around gluten. For some, this includes avoiding non–gluten-free bakeries. Flour particles are tiny and can stay suspended in the air for up to seventy-two hours; inhaling them may provoke a reaction. In your own home, keeping a hygienic kitchen is essential. To do this, follow the tips below:

- *Store any gluten-containing foods separately from your gluten-free foods.* Crumbs from bread, crackers, or cereal can contaminate gluten-free foods. Store gluten-free flours and baking mixes on the top shelf, where they cannot become contaminated from above. Wrapped frozen foods should be fine.
- You don't need to sterilize surfaces of pots and pans, nor do you need

a separate set of dishes or flatware. *Thorough washing with hot water and dish soap is adequate for most purposes*, except for a pasta pot and strainer (see below).

- *Avoid contaminating butter, margarine, peanut butter, jam, etc., with crumbs from non–gluten-free breads and baked goods.* Keep separate and labeled. Many gluten-free kitchens keep separate toasters for gluten-containing foods and gluten-free foods.

- *Designate a cutting board and storage area for your gluten-free bread and other foods.* A small waffle iron is also a wonderful, inexpensive addition to your kitchen. Label it "gluten-free," so you don't end up with crumbs of gluten-containing waffles in its crevices.

- *Always label (and date) leftovers.* I have accidentally eaten gluten this way, when there were two batches of noodles in the refrigerator, and someone ate my leftover rice pasta, leaving the semolina pasta in the same spot in an identical container.

- It is a good idea to *buy or designate one pot as your pasta pot*, because pasta tends to leave a film of starch on the pot unless very thoroughly washed. Some people tend to just rinse pasta pots and put them away, which could easily result in contamination of your gluten-free pasta from previously cooked wheat pasta.

- Since you may be the only one eating your gluten-free bread, and it has a short shelf life, *defrost only a few slices at a time.* Or take your morning bagel out the night before and let it thaw at room temperature. You'll waste less, and your baked goods will be more fresh.

- *Having recipes for your staple food products, and a shopping list that is specific for your gluten-free needs can be very helpful.* I felt well on my way after having good results with (1) a waffle recipe, (2) a pancake and crepe recipe, and (3) a muffin recipe. These are foods I eat often and would really miss if I couldn't make a gluten-free version.

Baking Mixes

I make up my own gluten-free flour mixes and baking mixes. In humid climates, they can become soggy and heavy unless you bake large quantities often. It might be better to make up baking mix as you go, from sealed packages of gluten-free flours. I keep a tightly sealed Tupperware containing my gluten-free mix in the refrigerator or freezer. Brown rice flour and some other flours can become rancid and off-tasting if not kept fresh. For many years, I have relied on the following very simple and reliable mix for quick-breads, pancakes, waffles, and crepes:

2 parts Bob's Red Mill Brown Rice Flour (or combine brown and white rice flours)

1 part Bob's Red Mill Sweet White Sorghum Flour

1 part Bob's Red Mill Tapioca Flour (or substitute part corn starch)

½ part Bob's Red Mill Potato Starch (not potato flour)

You can experiment with the basic baking mix by adding nut flours, like almond, hazelnut, or walnut meal (it is much less expensive to grind your own in a high speed blender); sweet rice flour, which is naturally sweet (available at Trader Joe's); or one of the more nutritious grains like quinoa, amaranth, or teff (available at Bob's Red Mill). For pancakes or waffles, try substituting pure buckwheat flour for ¼ to ⅓ of the flour mixture. Just be cautious that you are not buying buckwheat pancake and waffle mix, which contains gluten. Create your own style to suit your own taste.

I bake with eggs, and many of my products generally hold together well enough without adding xanthan or guar gums. However, if you want a product that holds together well, for example a coffee cake that you want to cut into squares before serving, you can add ½ teaspoon xanthan or guar gum per cup of flour mix to take the place of gluten. For breads and pizza crust, you may need to increase that to 1 teaspoon xanthan or guar gum to 1 cup of flour mix. Be sure to follow recipe directions for mixing times in order to distribute and develop the gum properly.

A word of caution about gums. Xanthan gum and guar gum are the two most popular gums or gluten substitutes used in gluten-free baking. Each has its place. *However, some people are sensitive to xanthan gum, occasionally highly sensitive. Unfortunately, their symptoms are gastrointestinal and can mimic a gluten exposure, with severe diarrhea, gas, and bloating.* Others just tend to have more frequent stools.

Guar gum tends to cause another issue. It actually acts as a bulk-forming laxative, similar to Metamucil or psyllium powder. While this can be a boon to those who tend to suffer constipation on a typical gluten-free diet high in white rice and rice flour, it can be a bit of an adjustment for others. I am sensitive to xanthan gum and prefer guar gum. Guar gum is also about half the price of xanthan gum. Both can usually be found in your grocery baking section, the gluten-free section, or in a specialty store.

Earth Balance Natural Buttery Spread is a good choice for baking or general use. It is vegan, lactose and gluten-free, and contains no trans-fats, but it does contain soy. Earth Balance is available in sticks for baking or in a plastic tub for everyday use.

Cookbook References

There has recently been an explosion in wonderful, nutritious gluten-free cooking, and many great cookbooks are coming onto the market. Some of my favorites include: *Sweet Alternatives: 100 Recipes Without Gluten, Dairy, or Sugar*, by Ariana Bundy; *Gluten-Free, Sugar-Free Cooking*, by Susan O'Brien; and the beautifully illustrated *Cooking Gluten-Free*, by Karen Robertson. See the Resources for additional information on following a gluten-free diet.

Gentle Herbal Remedies for Healing the Bladder and the Adrenals

Although there are other powerful medicinal herbs from Ayurvedic and Chinese medicinal traditions, some really require the direction and supervision of a skilled medical practitioner. Even many of our traditional Western medicinal herbs are too powerful to include in this guide for self-treatment. The herbs included here are all generally considered safe, unless specific cautions are mentioned. However, *some people may experience an unfavorable reaction to any one of them, so treat with caution.* Try a weak brew in a small amount the first few times to be sure you can tolerate it without any unwanted effects.

Please do not doubt that herbs are medicines! That being said, these are closer to over-the-counter than to prescription medicines, and I have tried to include cautionary information where warranted. Herbal medicine, while practiced worldwide for thousands of years, is *not* a substitute for good medical care, particularly in cases of infection. *A urinary tract infection can escalate to a kidney infection or sepsis and become life-threatening.* The herbs described here are best used to treat ongoing, chronic conditions. In some cases, if you find the right combination and dose, you may be able to wean off your prescription medication, but this should be done with the help and knowledge of your medical practitioner, and with the guidance of a skilled naturopathic physician or herbalist. *As with other medicines, always use the smallest effective dose possible.*

As with all medicines, inform your physician if you consistently take any herbs or supplements, as they may interact with medications or have other health consequences. *Never use herbal remedies when pregnant or nursing* except under the direction of a skilled herbalist. For a more comprehensive look at the benefits and possible side effects of herbal remedies, I recommend the book *Prescription or Poison?* by Amitava Dasgupta, PhD. The author provides a thorough, balanced overview of the uses of herbs and homeopathic remedies, and explains how herbs can interact with common medications, a point that is often overlooked.

To make a tea from any of these remedies, simply steep the desired amount of herb in water brought to a simmer for two to five minutes. In general, herbal remedies made from leaves require fewer minutes of steeping than those made from roots. I have made an effort to note which part of the plant is useful, or contains the desired medicinal properties.

Herbs for the Bladder

The following herbs, which are listed alphabetically, have a proven history of successful anecdotal use for treating bladder symptoms.

Birch Leaf (*Betula pendula*)

This remedy comes from the dried leaves of the silver birch, common in the British Isles, Europe, and Asia, but also used in North America as a landscape plant. It is a tall deciduous tree with golden fall color. Birch leaves have long been used as a treatment for both urinary symptoms and as a general pain tonic for arthritic symptoms. They have a slightly bitter taste when dried, but when mixed with other, more-flavorful herbs, the taste isn't noticeable, and you don't need to use many leaves to get a good medicinal effect. Birch leaves are a mild diuretic and contain disinfectant properties. They work well in conjunction with linden flower, described below. Birch leaf is probably only available as a dried herb in an herb shop. Or if you are lucky enough to have a tree in your yard, give it a try. Use just a few leaves at a time until you arrive at a brew that doesn't taste too bitter, but still has the pain-relieving action you require.

Chamomile (*Chamomilla recutita*)/German Chamomile (*Matricaria chamomilla*)

This mild herb has a pleasant, sweet taste, making it useful as a flavored herbal tea. The medicinal effects of chamomile flowers include the following: anti-inflammatory, antiseptic/antibiotic, sedative (mild), and antispasmodic properties. It is useful in treating indigestion, urinary tract symptoms, insomnia, and general nervousness. It is important to know that chamomile acts not only on the urinary tract but also relaxes the esophageal sphincter, so it isn't useful for conditions such as gastroesophageal reflex, or heartburn. Especially don't drink chamomile tea just before lying down, as it may cause acid reflux, even if you don't normally suffer this problem. Chamomile is useful to drink before a long car ride, however, or during a long family dinner, as it can help prevent the annoy-ing spasms that require frequent trips to the bathroom. Chamomile is safe for children's ailments in small amounts and has been relied on for its abil-ity to reduce fever quickly. In addition, chamomile has some antifungal action.

Cleavers (*Galium aparine*)/Lady's Bedstraw, or Yellow Bedstraw (*Galium verum*)

Cleavers, which is *Galium aparine*, and the related *Galium verum* are both used to treat kidney and urinary disorders, and they can also be used externally to treat wounds, skin rashes, and ulcerous conditions. When grown in your garden, the sweet-smelling white or pale cream-colored flowers are honey scented and the whole plant, whether fresh or dried, gives off a sweet, calming aroma. Cleavers has diuretic and urinary an-tiseptic properties and may help to prevent kidney stones. It should be avoided before bedtime.

Corn Silk (*Zea mays*)

The herbal remedy corn silk is the long strands or beard at the end of the corn cob. Corn silk makes a soothing diuretic for urinary tract symptoms and can help to ease the passage of urinary gravel and stones. Some people are very sensitive to the action of diuretics and should use them with cau-tion. Diuretics can lower blood pressure. Another property of corn silk is that it is a urinary demulcent, similar in action to marshmallow root, so it is a worthy substitute if other demulcent herbs don't agree with you. Avoid before bedtime.

Couch Grass (*Agropyron repens, Elytrigia repens*)

This common grass has long been used in Europe, where it is native, as a gentle cure for urinary tract symptoms. The rhizomes, or long, under-ground runners, are the medicinally useful part of the plant. When dried, they have a mild pleasant taste and the following medicinal properties: an-tiseptic/antimicrobial, mild diuretic, anti-inflammatory, and mucilage, all of which make couch grass useful for soothing inflamed bladders. It has also been used to treat gout, rheumatism, prostate problems, and bladder stones. You can find this herb in an herb shop, or in powdered, capsule form in the supplements section of a natural foods store or pharmacy.

Cramp Bark (*Viburnum opulus*)

Viburnum contains a plant sterol that acts as a phytoestrogen. It is useful as an antispasmodic for the female genitourinary tract and it has some anti-inflammatory properties. Cramp bark is a strong herb, but I'm including it here because it is one of the best treatments for both menstrual cramps and mid-cycle ovarian pain. Because it is an excellent relaxant, it is also useful for alleviating muscle cramps in general. *Avoid this plant if you take Coumadin (or other blood thinners) or have a platelet disorder, and never use this plant if you are pregnant or nursing*, unless under the care of a highly skilled herbalist.

Fennel Seed (*Foeniculum vulgare*)
Fennel seeds have been used since the Middle Ages for their digestive properties and to freshen the breath. The seeds contain linoleic acid, bioflavonoids, vitamins, and minerals. Fennel also has some phytoestrogenic properties. Medicinally the seeds are used to treat indigestion, heartburn, colic, gas, and bloating. They are known to have antispasmodic, anti-inflammatory and antibacterial properties. Fennel seeds have a pleasant, licorice-like taste. The best way to use fennel seed is to crush it slightly with a mortar and pestle and then add it to other herbal ingredients, steep the mixture in hot/boiling water for 3–5 minutes, and then strain to produce a hot, pleasant tea that will ease your digestive difficulties. The seeds can also be used to flavor certain foods, like pizza sauce, sausages, and minestrone soup.

Goldenrod (*Solidago canadensis*)
Goldenrod is known primarily as a cleansing herb. It is also a beautiful native wildflower, with a plume of golden flowers in early fall. The flowering tips and leaves are used to brew a tea that is useful in treating urinary infections. It may also help to relieve lower back pain referred from the bladder or pain from arthritis, although that isn't its primary use. Goldenrod has a cleansing action specifically on mucous membranes. I would consider goldenrod for active infection, along with concurrent medical treatment, but not for those with fragile bladder linings, as these people need all the protective mucous they can hold onto. In addition, *if you suffer from a chronic kidney disorder, goldenrod should be used cautiously and under the care of a skilled herbalist.*

Lemon Balm (Melissa; *Melissa officinalis*)
Lemon balm is a very easy-to-grow member of the mint family. Like any mint, it can even be a garden pest if not maintained, but its pleasant, lemony scent, lime-green leaves, and multiple uses outweigh that consideration, in my opinion. (One caveat is that if you live near a natural area, you may want to avoid growing this herb, which can easily escape cultivation

and become a problem.) The leaves are used medicinally, and they produce a very pleasant hot or cold tea with a delicate lemon flavor. Besides having antispasmodic properties that make it useful for digestive problems, lemon balm has a wonderful combination of both calming and uplifting properties. It is helpful for tension headaches, general pain and discomfort, depression, sadness, nervousness, anxiety, and insomnia. It also has antihistamine, antispasmodic, antiviral, antibacterial, and relaxant properties, so it can substitute for many other herbs. If you're out of nettle leaf and need an antihistamine, lemon balm is a good second choice. If your bladder is highly inflamed, though, the essential oils contained in lemon balm — citral, geraniol, citronellal, and the tannins — can cause mild irritation, especially if the tea is strongly brewed. A few leaves in another, more soothing mixture may be tolerated. Due to its unique pleasant taste, a few leaves of this herb can be used to flavor other mixtures. If mosquitoes or gnats are bothering you, crush a few fresh leaves of lemon balm to release their essential oils, and rub gently over your skin as a repellant. You can find lemon balm in a dried form, but it loses its essential oils and medicinal properties more quickly than many dried herbs and is much more effective and tasty when fresh.

Linden Flower (*Tilia europaea, Tilia cordata, Tilia platyphyllos*)

Linden, or "lime," trees are tall, graceful shade trees with a wide canopy of dark green, heart-shaped leaves. Although native and common in Europe and the British Isles, they are also a common street tree now in North America. The flowering arrangement on this species is very unique, being attached to the leaves by a flattened stalk, which makes it very easy to identify. The flowers are tiny and pale cream-colored, and they are among the most delightfully scented flowers I know. I would definitely go out of my way to walk under a canopy of lime trees in full flower on a warm summer night! The medicinal compounds of these sweet-smelling flowers include hesperidin and quercetin bioflavonoids (which may help to lower blood pressure), the mineral manganese, and mucilaginous properties, which may help to soothe the bladder. Mucilaginous herbs contain special starches that produce a mucouslike coating in the urinary tract. It is a mild diuretic, which makes it useful to drink after dinner, but not right before bedtime. Other components of this herb are antispasmodic, and it seems to be particularly useful in calming a restless bladder, preventing bladder spasms, and producing a good flow of urine. *I personally recommend linden as one of the best herbs for the bladder, even though this use isn't especially well known here in the United States.*

Hot tea made from lime flowers helps to relax the nervous system and enhance sleep, relieve headaches, and treat insomnia. Like chamomile, lime flower is considered a safe remedy for reducing fevers in children, as long as they are well-hydrated. *Anytime a fever exists, adequate fluid intake is essential, and losing fluids through the diuretic action of herbal remedies or through diarrhea, excessive sweating, or vomiting makes the situation worse. Always try to get the person to drink fluids and, if they can't keep them down, seek medical attention immediately.* One caveat is that it is sometimes difficult to find lime flowers, and linden leaves, although pleasant tasting, do not have the same medicinal effect on the bladder.

Marshmallow Root (*Althaea officinalis*)

Native to the British Isles, marshmallow is a perennial herb with light pink flowers that is commonly found in salt marshes and other moist places. The entire plant can be used medicinally, but the root is traditionally used to treat bladder and intestinal disorders, including cystitis, urethritis, and gastroenteritis. Marshmallow root is one of the most important mucilaginous herbs, helping to protectively coat and sooth irritated mucous membranes. Marshmallow root is also anti-inflammatory and mildly diuretic. It is considered to be a demulcent herb—a remedy used to soothe the respiratory, digestive, and urinary systems. This herbal remedy seems to be most soothing when brewed as a tea, strained, and allowed to cool to room temperature. It should have a slightly sticky, thickened, although clear, appearance due to its high mucilage content. Marshmallow is also available in an herbal capsule, although used in this way it isn't as effective for bladder symptoms. In my experience, marshmallow root can sometimes be contaminated with mold, and it is high in oxalates, so it may not be a good remedy for everyone, despite its popularity for use in IC treatment.

Nettle Leaf (*Urtica dioica*)

Nettle is a perennial herb with many medicinal properties. The common name is "stinging nettle," because of the many fine stinging hairs which release formic acid when touched. Be careful when hiking in areas where it grows as it reaches about to fingertip height, and a swing of the arms can bring your fingers into contact with the leaves (and you will soon find out how it got its name).

The flowering stems and leaves contain this plant's abundant medicinal properties. Nettle leaf has astringent, tonic, and diuretic properties. Nettle is one of the best—if not the best—natural antihistamines, and it is also a good anti-inflammatory. Both of these properties make it very useful in treating bladder disorders, and *I personally recommend nettle leaf highly as an herb for the bladder, particularly for those with food sensi-tivities and allergies.* Another unique property of the plant is its nutrient content. Nettle leaves are full of vitamins A and C and minerals such as iron, manganese, silica, and sulfur. It is a very good remedy for anemia. However, nettle can be a very strong herb, and it is also high in potassium, which could possibly irritate some people with IC. A little nettle goes a long way—it isn't necessary to brew a strong tea—and you'll receive the medicinal benefit even from a very weak brew. Nettle is also a powerful "green" plant and a good source of chlorophyll, which helps to alkalinize the body (red clover and alfalfa are also alkalizing herbs for the bladder). So, what about those stinging hairs? They are rendered harmless when the plant is cooked like spinach or brewed into a tea.

No doubt due to its antihistamine effect, I have noticed that applying some of the tea to a skin irritation quickly resolves the itch.

Nettle leaf teas are manufactured by several companies, and nettle leaf is nearly always available as a bulk dried herb in natural-foods stores, as it is one of our most valuable and commonly used medicinal herbs. If try-ing to harvest and dry your own, simply wear a pair of leather gardening gloves and put the clipped flowering stems in a large brown paper bag to transport home. However, it is extremely important to *only harvest nettle leaves early in the spring* when the leaves are newly formed. Mature nettle leaves can contain substances that can actually cause urinary tract irrita-tion.

Stinging-nettle "root" is a remedy distinct from nettle leaf that has shown some usefulness in treating prostate inflammation (BPH), some-times in combination with saw palmetto. These are both anti-inflamma-tory herbs, and they help to balance one another.

Pipsissewa (*Chimaphila umbellate* and *Chimaphila menziesii*)

This member of the wintergreen family grows in the dark forests of the Pacific Northwest on humus or rotting wood. It is a little fairy plant with a creeping rhizome; nodding pinkish-white, waxy flowers; and whorled evergreen leaves. The leaves contain medicinal properties and have been brewed into tea by many native peoples to treat everything from colds and influenza to kidney stones. Pipsissewa is different from the other herbs discussed previously because it has shown itself to have an *antidiuretic* ef-fect in experiments. This probably means you should not use this plant if you suffer from congestive heart failure, high blood pressure, or fluid re-tention. Pipsissewa is related to uva-ursi (bearberry) but is lower in tan-nins and less harsh, so it can be used in nonacute situations. The leaves have a slightly bitter taste and should be used in small quantities in conjunction with other teas. However, the leaves aren't as distasteful as many bitter herbs, so you shouldn't be afraid to give pipsissewa a try. It is sometimes available as a dried herb in capsule form.

Peppermint (*Mentha piperita*)

Peppermint is an easy-to-grow perennial herb, and, in fact, it sometimes escapes cultivation to become a nuisance. Many people are very familiar with peppermint as a culinary herb and a flavorful beverage, but peppermint does have medicinal effects as well. When I worked on a busy hospital surgical floor I found that peppermint tea has a stimulatory effect on the digestive system, helping to promote a return to normal bowel activity, stimulating the flow of bile, and relieving gas pain. Peppermint also has antispasmodic properties (especially for the smooth muscles), mild anesthetic properties, and antibacterial properties, all of which make it useful for helping to alleviate bladder and bowel symptoms. It also has some anti-inflammatory properties. When brewed too long, peppermint can become harsh and slightly bitter due to its high tannin content, and the flavor can be overwhelming. Steep your peppermint tea only briefly, or combine it with other herbs to add a bit of flavor. Peppermint combines well with other herbs in mixtures used to treat the stomach, bladder, and respiratory system. In general, peppermint is probably much more useful in treating irritable bowel syndrome (IBS) than in treating IC. The IC bladder may be too sensitive to tolerate peppermint.

Plantain (*Plantago lanceolata*)

Plantain is a common perennial herb with prostrate leaves that have parallel veins, like a grass. The leaves are used medicinally as a mucilaginous herb with emollient, demulcent, and astringent, or cleansing, properties that make it useful for treating wounds and general irritations of the mucous membranes. Thus, it is useful for treating irritated bladders and for bronchitis, coughs, hoarseness, and general respiratory symptoms. Plantain is also antibacterial and anti-inflammatory. It is usually available in capsule form and as a dried herb, but plantain is also a very common lawn weed and is easily recognized. If using the fresh plant, make sure it comes from an organic, herbicide-free source. The seeds are used as a bulk laxative. You may have heard of psyllium, which is from a related plant, *Plantago psyllium*.

Pygeum (*Pygeum africanum*)

I've been reading a lot about this herb recently, especially regarding its use in treating prostate inflammation. Pygeum is widely used in Europe, and a number of substantive clinical studies have shown its usefulness in reducing swelling in the prostate. This makes it a useful herb for treating both BPH and chronic prostatitis. Pygeum may also have some anticancer benefit. This remedy is found most commonly as a tincture or liquid extract. It comes from the bark of a tree in Africa, and there is a potential for overharvesting. Saw palmetto or nettle root would make a good substitute.

Red Raspberry Leaf (*Rubus idaeus*)

Red raspberry leaf is commonly available if you know anyone who grows raspberries in their garden. It is great to brew a tea from fresh leaves, especially in the spring, and it is very easy to harvest and dry. It is tasty and retains its medicinal effects whether fresh or dry. Red raspberry leaf has been used to treat women's ailments for thousands of years, with one caveat: *It contains oxytoxic properties, meaning it can make the uterus contract. It should not be used during pregnancy without the specific administration of a trained nurse-midwife.*

I first discovered the healing and comforting properties of red raspberry leaf when treating myself for uncomfortable menstrual cramps. I grew to depend on this gentle herb from my home garden to ease discomfort at the start of my period. I also really enjoy the taste. Red raspberries (fruits) are good sources of both iron and vitamin C, and this enhances the absorption of the iron. For inflammatory conditions such as endometriosis, red raspberry leaf is useful, especially when combined with hormone-balancing herbs such as vitex (chasteberry).

Red raspberry leaf is available in a tea-bag form from many manufacturers, but be sure to try it fresh if you have access to it. That's not at all difficult in the Pacific Northwest, where I live.

Rooibos/Redbush (*Aspalathus linearis*)

Redbush tea, or rooibos tea, is made from a shrubby member of the legume family native to the mountains of South Africa. The tasty beverage brewed from the leaves of the redbush plant has a good reputation for promoting health. Much of its health benefit is due to its very high antioxidant content, which helps to protect the body from ongoing oxidative stress. It is particularly useful in protecting the eyes and other mucous membranes from damage and in preventing vascular complications in diabetics. (It also helps to regulate blood sugar.) This flavorful herb may be helpful for those with bladder issues because it has anti-inflammatory and antispasmodic effects, helps to lower histamine levels and control the allergenic response, and may even help with sleep. Redbush is of special use as an alternative beverage for those with IC, because it is low in tannins and contains no caffeine. Redbush tea is a better source of minerals than regular black or green tea, and it is calorie-free. The sweet, nutty taste of redbush tea can be enjoyed hot or cold, with milk or without. You'll be glad you gave this delicious tea a try. Look for tea bags and bulk loose tea in your grocery or natural-foods store.

Saw Palmetto (*Serenoa repens* or *Sabal serrulata*)

Saw palmetto is well known for its use in treating inflammation of the prostate in men and is widely available. The berries and their constituents are used medicinally. Regular use of this remedy aids in urination, and so helps to prevent the consequences of urine retention, namely urinary tract infection. Some sources also recommend saw palmetto for low libido, low testosterone, and impotence. This remedy may also be useful to women with infertility or hormonal imbalances associated with painful periods. The berries have a soothing quality on mucous membranes, and have a mildly sedating affect on the nervous system. Overall, its traditional use is to treat urinary disorders that include a difficulty or inability to void.

Slippery Elm (*Ulmus fulva*)

Slippery elm has long been used to treat inflammation and to sooth irritations involving the mucous membranes of the gastrointestinal tract. The dried inner bark contains the mucilaginous properties that this herb is known for. Slippery elm infusions (teas) and slippery elm gruel (the powdered form of the herb mixed into a paste with hot water) help to lubricate and soothe mucous membranes, relieve inflammation, and treat diarrhea. These remedies are considered safe enough for children.

Because it is the inner bark that contains the medicinal properties, make sure that is what you are getting, and not the coarse outer bark, which does not contain these properties. Use this amazing healing remedy if you need it, but be aware that it is in short supply and collection of the inner bark usually leads to the trees' destruction. Marshmallow root or linden flower are good alternatives.

Vitex (Chasteberry, Monk's Pepper; *Vitex agnus-castus*)

Even the name suggests its medicinal action as a hormone balancer. The fruit, or berry, is used medicinally. It helps to regulate estrogen and progesterone production, and, as such, is useful for treating endometriosis, premenstrual tension, and excessive menstrual bleeding. It also has been shown in laboratory and clinical studies to increase the production of prolactin, increasing the flow of breast milk. It is inexpensive and widely available in capsule form, and it is included in several combination remedies for both PMS and menopause relief. I personally recommend chasteberry for helping to relieve menopausal symptoms and balance a woman's estrogen-to-progesterone balance.

White Willow Bark (*Salix alba*)

White willow bark has three main medicinal properties: It is an anti-inflammatory, with a particular effect on the joints; it reduces fevers; and it helps to reduce pain. Willow and its relatives are a natural source of salicylic acid, the chemical compound in aspirin. Unlike aspirin, it does not easily irritate the stomach, and it has, in fact, been used to treat stomach ailments. The dried bark, which is used medicinally in teas and tinctures, has a bitter taste, but it is quite palatable when mixed with milder herbs. It is very effective for nerve pain and headaches, and it may help to reduce the severe pain of a bladder condition. White willow bark should not be used long-term, but it can be a short-term fix until you reach medical attention.

Wild Yam (*Dioscorea villosa*)

Wild yam is a tropical vine common in the southeastern United States. It isn't the same plant as Mexican yam or Mexican wild yam, so it is important to buy it from a reputable supplier to ensure that you are getting the correct product. Although some women's formulas contain this herb and its marketing has been confusing, wild yam contains no hormone precursors. According to noted herbalist Michael Moore, "[W]ild yam is a preeminent smooth muscle relaxant and antispasmodic herb…PERIOD." But, that's still good news for us. Available in tincture or capsule form, wild yam may be a good herb to keep on hand for menstrual cramps, bladder or urethral spasms, and crampy bowel pains. Wild yam also contains anti-inflammatory properties, and it has even been used to treat rheumatoid arthritis. Another species of the same genus, *D. mexicana,* has been used to synthesize progesterone for use in contraceptives.

Wild yam has a diuretic effect, so use it cautiously if frequency is a problem for you and be sure to avoid taking it just before going to bed.

Herbs for Adrenal Health

The following herbs have been suggested by many sources as useful tools in promoting adrenal health and in facilitating recovery from adrenal fatigue.

Astragalus (*Astragalus membranaceus*)

Astragalus is an important herb in traditional Chinese medicine (TCM) and is considered an adaptogen, an herb that helps the body move toward balance. For instance, an adaptogen will take on different characteristics depending on whether the action required is stimulating or calming. The dried root is used to strengthen the immune system and improve adrenal gland function. Through its anti-inflammatory, immune-boosting, and antioxidant effects, astragalus can be used in cases of multiple allergies, chronic fatigue, anemia, and general digestive issues. Astragalus does have diuretic effects, so it may increase the action of prescription diuretics. Astragalus should also be used with caution if a patient is taking immunosuppressant medications, anticoagulants, or medications used to treat blood sugar and blood pressure. This herb should not be used in cases of fever. Of special interest is that astragalus has been used in treating painful urination and kidney inflammation, and that it improves the flow of urine. In general this herb is well-tolerated by the bladder, and may be a good choice for those who cannot tolerate ginseng, which is often suggested for cases of adrenal fatigue.

Ashwagandha Root (*Withania somnifera*)

Many physicians and herbalists consider ashwagandha to be one of the most important herbs for recovery from adrenal fatigue, and *I recommend it highly for treatment of adrenal fatigue and bladder issues.*

Ashwagandha is an important herb in Ayurvedic medicine (India's ancient medicinal tradition). It has many medicinal properties, and it is considered to be an adaptogen. Ashwagandha is known for its anti-inflammatory action and its ability as a tonic that supports the adrenals. It can be combined with other herbs that support adrenal health into a tea blend, or it can be taken as an herbal capsule. Ashwagandha seems to have a relaxing, antispasmodic affect on the bladder, but not so much that it causes urinary hesitancy — in fact, it seems to help relieve urinary hesitancy and normalize voiding function, helping to improve the flow of urine. Overall, it is a great herb for the bladder, whether you have overactive bladder or IC.

Borage Leaf (*Borago officinalis*)

Borage is a common garden herb with bright blue flowers. It is related to comfrey, another healing plant, and is native to Europe. The leaves are generally used as a gentle remedy for balancing and restoring the adrenals and other endocrine glands. It is also anti-inflammatory, and it has been used successfully to treat skin conditions such as psoriasis and eczema.

Because borage leaves contain potassium and calcium, use them with caution if you are sensitive to potassium. Consider adding a pinch of this useful herb to other herbs in an adrenal-support blended tea — it combines well with nettle and linden. Borage can be used daily.

Ginger Root (*Zingiber officinale*)

Ginger root — the familiar root used frequently in Asian cooking, or dried, ground, and used as a spice for desserts — is also an important medicinal herb. Ginger root is useful for the adrenals because it helps modulate the stress-response hormone. Long known in the culinary world and in Ayurvedic medicine as an herb that stimulates digestion, ginger is great for alleviating nausea and morning sickness, too. Making ginger tea from the fresh root is very easy, and it is delicious with a little honey to sweeten it. In the past few years, it has become a more common ingredient in commercial tea preparations.

Gingko Leaf (*Gingko biloba*)

Gingko is a powerful free-radical scavenger, helping to protect the adrenal glands from oxidative stress, which can occur when the adrenals are forced to produce excess cortisol during the stress response. (Free radicals can start a cascade of cell-damaging effects, and antioxidants such as gingko are able to remove free radicals and inhibit damaging oxidation reactions in the body.) Gingko's ability to protect tissues from damage from free radicals makes it an important herb to use in cases of adrenal fatigue. Combined with gingko's well-known ability to sharpen mental acuity and help alleviate depression, this herb can contribute substantially to any recovery program addressing adrenal fatigue. Gingko is widely available in many forms.

Licorice Root (*Glycyrrhiza glabra*)

Licorice root is considered one of the most powerful and specific herbs for restoring the adrenals. Fortunately, licorice is also very tasty, is naturally sweet, and combines well with many other herbs. It can be overpowering for a sensitive IC bladder, and you may need to dilute it quite a bit in the beginning. Some people may not even be able to tolerate licorice root at all. Try buying the fresh dried root from a reputable herb source and brewing it to a light yellow color to produce a tea with a delicate licorice flavor. You can combine it with other herbs used to treat either the bladder or the adrenal glands.

Licorice root has a reputation for raising blood pressure and upsetting electrolyte balance if used too frequently. Many people with adrenal fatigue have unusually low blood pressure, so for most this might not be much of a problem. Licorice root is powerful, so it is not a good everyday herb, and certainly should not be used in strong or frequent doses or for a child (without the guidance of a skilled herbal practitioner). Using licorice root occasionally or several times a week may be a safe option, but it would be best to check with a qualified herbalist. Licorice root has soothing, anti-spasmodic, and laxative effects on the gastrointestinal system.

Rhodiola (*Rhodiola rosea*)

Rhodiola, also known as golden root, is native to the circumpolar regions. In both Siberian and Scandinavian folk medicine, rhodiola has been traditionally used to treat fatigue and depression. In herbal medicine, it is classified as an adaptogen. It has some unusual qualities that make it a good choice for treating adrenal fatigue: It can be used to calm emotional instability and emotional stress at the same time that it can help to energize and support the cognitive function. Rhodiola is known to enhance cellular energy metabolism, which is useful for treating cases of fatigue. Look for it in capsule form from a reliable supplier. Rhodiola is well thought of by many naturopaths who treat those with adrenal fatigue.

Siberian Ginseng (*Eleuthera ginseng*)

This powerful restorative herb isn't closely related to the harsher Chinese ginseng, or Panax ginseng, although it shares some of the same qualities. In general, this is the gentler herb, and the one that is a better choice for women. Many naturopaths speak highly of Eleuthera as an herb well-suited for treating cases of adrenal fatigue and for hormone balancing in general. It can be combined with other herbs for stimulating and balancing the adrenals. I cannot personally recommend this herb, as my bladder, which is well-healed, did not seem to do well with it, but it is highly recommended by many other people, so it might be worth a try if you're suffering from adrenal fatigue.

Purchasing Herbs

If you don't have access to a good herb store in your part of the country, consider ordering from the following sources:

Avena Botanicals
219 Mill St., Rockport ME 04856
(207) 594-0694   www.avenabotanicals.com
Avena is one of the nation's largest suppliers of herbs.

Great Cape Herbs
P.O. Box 1206, Brewster MA 02631
(800) 427-7144   www.greatcape.com

Mountain Rose Herbs
P.O. Box 50220, Eugene OR 97405
(800) 879-3337   info@mountainroseherbs.com
www.mountainroseherbs.com
A reliable source for organic dried herbs of consistent quality.

Oregon's Wild Harvest
Sandy OR
(800) 316-6869   www.oregonswildharvest.com

Penn Herb Company, Ltd.
10601 Decatur Rd., Philadelphia PA 19154
(800) 523-9971   http://pennherb.com/index.html

There are hundreds of good books on herbal medicine, many available at your local library. I have drawn information from my undergraduate studies in botany and many years of personal experience. I have verified this information using a variety of books and other sources, including those listed below:

Bunney, S., ed., *The Illustrated Encyclopedia of Herbs — Their Medicinal and Culinary Uses*. Prague, Czech Republic: Aventinum, 1984.

Fetrow, C. W., and J. R. Avila. *The Complete Guide to Herbal Medicines*. New York: Pocket Books, 2000.

Gagnier, J. J., M. W. Van Tulder, B. Berman, and C. Bombadier. "Herbal Medicine for Low Back Pain: A Cochrane Review." *Spine* 32 (2007): 82–92.

Mabey, R., ed. *The New Age Herbalist — How to Use Herbs for Healing, Nutrition, Body Care, and Relaxation*. New York: Collier Books, 1988.

McIntyre, A. *Herbs for Common Ailments*. New York: Simon & Schuster — Fireside Books, 1992.

Moore, M. "Interstitial Cystitis — An Herbal Approach." http://www .scribd.com/doc/14881293/Interstitial-Cystitis-An-Herbal-Approach (accessed 14 October 2009).

Moore, M. *Herbs for the Urinary Tract*. New York: McGraw-Hill, 1999.

Phaneuf, H. *Herbs Demystified: A Scientist Explains How the Most Common Herbal Remedies Really Work*. Cambridge, MA: DaCapo Press, 2005.

Pojar, J., and A. MacKinnon. *Plants of the Pacific Northwest Coast— Washington, Oregon, British Columbia & Alaska.* Auburn, WA: Ministry of Forests and Lone Pine Publishing, 1994.

Tilgner, S. *Herbal Medicine—From the Heart of the Earth.* 2nd ed. Cresswell, OR: Wise Acres Press, 2009.

Homeopathic Remedies for the Bladder

Homeopathic remedies can be used in two ways—first, as constitutional remedies, and second, as remedies to treat specific complaints. Homeopathy is a science unto itself, and well beyond the scope of this book. However, since homeopathy can provide relief and isn't expensive, it is worth a try when you're really suffering. Some women have had good results using homeopathy under the guidance of a practicing homeopath.

The science of homeopathy was developed over 150 years ago by a German physician, and became popular in Europe and then North America. Homeopathy uses very dilute remedies made from natural substances: plants, minerals, and even some derived from animals. Homeopathy is based on the principle of "like treats like." To the Western-trained mind it often doesn't make much sense. But homeopathy has a long track record of some success, is inexpensive, nontoxic, and often a single remedy is effective.

A Guide to Using Homeopathic Remedies

When selecting homeopathic remedies, you will see that the name of a remedy is followed by a number and a letter, as in "Cantharis 30C." This "30C" denotes the dilution factor. Homeopathic remedies are highly diluted natural substances, and in what seems contrary to our Western minds, the more diluted the remedy, the stronger it is. For example, 30C remedy, although diluted many more times, is stronger than a 6C remedy. Remedies can also contain the letters X and M, which are much stronger, and these should be used only with the guidance of a homeopathic or naturopathic physician.

You can make an appointment to see a qualified homeopath, or a naturopath who is also specially trained in homeopathy. However, Boiron makes a line of over-the-counter homeopathic remedies for common ailments, and some of these may be applicable to your situation. You may find these in your natural-foods store or natural pharmacy. They are inexpensive, generally cause no harm, and come in lower dosages, usually from 6C to 30C. Be aware that most homeopathic remedies are made with a base of lactose, or milk sugar. *If you are very sensitive to lactose, even the minor amount contained in the tiny pellets can make you have loose stools and suffer abdominal cramping.*

Some women on IC website forums have had good experiences with some of the following remedies, and I have also had some symptomatic relief from several of these recommended remedies.

Two good general references for using homeopathic remedies are the following:

Griffith, C. *The Practical Handbook of Homeopathy.* Winchester, UK: Baird, Duncan Publishers, 2008.

Panos, M. B., and J. Heimlich. *Homeopathic Medicine at Home — Natural Remedies for Everyday Ailments and Minor Injuries.* New York: Tarcher Penguin Books, 1990.

Apis

The Apis remedy is a good choice when the patient is irritable and experiences stinging pain as the urine passes through the urethra. The urethra itself may feel swollen and irritated.

Belladonna

Belladonna works on the nervous system, including neuropathic pain that comes and goes, throbbing pain, bladder pain and inflammation, painful or difficult urination, urgency, nocturia, restless sleep, and bladder spasms.

Berberis Vulgaris

This remedy is useful for arthritic symptoms accompanied by urinary symptoms, including wandering, radiating pains. Berberis is specifically for people who have increased pain on standing or when standing brings on urinary complaints. Other urinary complaints for which Berberis is useful include sudden, sharp, stinging pain; pain leading into the urethra; bladder pain; tearing around the anus; and a sensation of incomplete bladder emptying.

Cantharis

Use this remedy for interstitial cystitis or bladder infection when accompanied by burning pain and pain with urination. Conditions that can be helped by cantharis include bladder pain brought on by drinking coffee, pain with or difficulty urinating, constant urge to urinate, scanty urine containing blood or pus, urine retention, and urinary hesitancy. Patient may feel pain and tenderness in the lower abdomen/pelvis, as if the intestines are inflamed. Symptoms may be accompanied by anxiety and restlessness.

Copaiva Officinalis
This remedy acts powerfully on mucous membranes, especially the urinary tract. Conditions that Copaiva may help include urinary hesitancy and urine retention, difficulty starting a stream, a thin urine stream, spasmodic bladder pain, and urinary frequency. Other conditions for which Copaiva may be helpful include chronic urticaria (hives) and itching of the vulva and anus. Persons for whom this remedy may be helpful are sensitive to sharp sounds and sometimes complain of pain in the occiput (back of the skull).

Pulsatilla Nigricans
Traditionally, Pulsatilla is useful for people with gentle, weepy dispositions and those who are highly emotional. It is used to treat bladder inflammation, urgency, hesitancy, frequency, dribbling, and interrupted or intermittent voiding. It is also useful for treating women who have abdominal/pelvic heaviness and crampy pain before and during their periods. (This seems like it would be a good remedy for treating the symptoms of endometriosis.)

People for whom this remedy is a good choice often have a lack of thirst, even though drinking cold drinks helps relieve their symptoms.

Sepia
Patients who respond to this remedy may feel heaviness and fullness in the pelvic area, and they may experience stress incontinence. Fatigue, irritability, and dysuria are common symptoms. This remedy is also used to treat headaches in women, specifically headaches that begin behind the left eye and migraine-type headaches in which the only thing people want to do is lie down in a darkened room.

Viburnum Opulus
This is a great homeopathic remedy that is specifically for the relief of one-sided ovarian pain at mid-cycle. I've never found anything else that works so well. It is more-generally useful for crampy pain in the pelvic organs, which can include the bladder, uterus, ovaries, and fallopian tubes.

*(**Diagnosis discussion** continued from page 38)*

Patients with IC also have greater levels of histamine and substance P (an inflammatory neurotransmitter) in their urine than non-IC patients. Elevated levels of histamine may indicate an allergic component to IC.

Another important finding is that the bladder epithelium of IC patients secretes a protein fragment called anti-proliferative factor (APF), which limits the body's natural mechanism for repairing the bladder lining. Scientists are actively engaged in determining the role of APF and understanding why it is produced in the bladders of IC patients. It remains an important factor in IC research and represents one of the best possibilities for developing a reliable "biomarker" specifically associated with IC.

Significantly, the new AUA guidelines suggest that hydrodistention with cystoscopy is not necessary or required for making the diagnosis of IC in routine cases but should be considered when needed to help rule out conditions such as bladder cancer. This "Expert Opinion" represents a significant shift from past clinical practices encouraging hydrodistention with cystoscopy, primarily because new evidence has found glomerulations on the bladder wall to be variable and possibly consistent with other bladder conditions. Patients may also be pleased to know that the potassium sensitivity test (PST) is no longer recommended for routine use in patients with typical symptoms of IC. The group determined the test does not help to exclude other disorders, rarely changes the treatment plan, is painful for patients, and can lead to increased symptoms.

In summary, if a patient has frequent urination and pain that increases with bladder filling and improves after urinating, the clinician can make the presumptive diagnosis of IC after excluding other disorders (as above). These new AUA guidelines for IC diagnosis and treatment will hopefully help to speed up the process of diagnosis and get patients into effective treatment more quickly.

NOTES

The Better Bladder Book is heavily researched and documented; therefore, the Notes are very lengthy. In an effort to have the book be reasonably priced and to conserve paper, the Notes can be found online at www.the betterbladderbookinfo.com. Professionals are welcome to contact me directly, either through the publisher or via any of my websites.

RESOURCES

Further Information and Support

Interstitial Cystitis (IC)

Books

Chalker, R., and K. Whitmore. *Overcoming Bladder Disorders*. New York: HarperCollins, 1990. *Although somewhat outdated now, it is a good general overview of IC and other urological disorders.*

Moldwin, R. M. *The Interstitial Cystitis Survival Guide: Your Guide to the Latest Treatment Options and Coping Strategies*. Oakland: New Harbinger Publications, 2000. *Written by a physician and IC patient, this book provides a compassionate, comprehensive look at IC, written mostly from a traditional allopathic medical perspective.*

Vliet, E. L. *Screaming to Be Heard: The Hormonal Connections Women Suspect and Doctors Still Ignore*. Rev. and exp. ed. New York: M. Evans and Company, 2001. *See especially Chapter 12: "Interstitial Cystitis, Vulvodynia, and Leaky Bladders" for an insightful discussion on IC and related topics.*

Willis, A. K. *Solving the Interstitial Cystitis Puzzle: A Guide to Natural Healing*. Rev. ed. Los Angeles, CA: Holistic Life Enterprises, 2003. *This book provides a wealth of information on the importance of following an alkaline diet for IC.*

Author's Note: With the exception of these four general references, I have relied primarily on my own review of a large number of peer-reviewed research studies and professional journal articles.

Articles

Kriz, R. "Bacteria and IC—But How Can That Be When My Urine Cultures Are All Negative?" Interstitial Cystitis Information Center. http://www.moonstar.com/~icickay/articles/bacteria_ic.pdf.

Sandler, G. "Surviving Painful Flare Ups." In *IC Lifestyles & Exercise—A Monthly Column on Lifestyle, Fitness, and Relationships.* IC Network, 2005. http://www.ic-network.com/iclifestyles/june05.html.

Organizations, Support Groups, and Websites

Interstitial Cystitis Association (ICA)
(800) HELP-ICA *or* (301) 610-5300
ICAmail@ichelp.org   www.ichelp.org

Interstitial Cystitis Network (ICN)
www.ic-network.com *and* www.ic-network.com/md
ICN MD list (MDs, counselors, physical therapists, dieticians, and IC specialists by region).

IC Puzzle (support group)
http://healthgroups.yahoo.com/group/icpuzzle
Online support group started by Amrit Willis, RN, author of Solving the Interstitial Cystitis Puzzle. *Most participants are interested in a holistic perspective.*

Interstitial Cystitis Support Group (ICSG), United Kingdom
+44.1908.569169
www.interstitialcystitis.co.uk   info@interstitialcystitis.co.uk

International Painful Bladder Foundation (IPBF)
www.painful-bladder.org *and*
www.painful-bladder.org/globalgroups_etc.html
This is a link to a comprehensive list of support groups worldwide in more than thirty countries.

National Kidney and Urological Diseases Information Clearinghouse
http://kidney.niddk.nih.gov/kudiseases/pubs/interstitialcystitis
Good information source on a variety of urological diseases, including IC.

Pure Hope (Pelvic and Urological Resources and Education)
www.pure-hope.org/index.htm
Support organization that sponsors an annual conference and acts as an information clearinghouse.

Urology Wellness Center
www.urologywellnesscenter.com

Information on B. J. Carapata, CRNP, CUNP, an important voice for complementary therapies for IC, particularly long-term antibiotic therapy.

The Urology Center of Colorado (TUCC)
2777 Mile High Stadium Cir., Denver CO 80211
(877) 825-8898
This large urology practice has an "IC team" that practices an interdisciplinary approach.

WellBladder
www.wellbladder.com
This is my website, and it contains information on a variety of IC and bladder-related topics, important articles, and links to resources.

❄ *For a Urine Broth Culture*

United Medical Lab
6720 Old McLean Village Dr., McLean VA 22101
(703) 356-4422   www.unitedmedicallabs.com
Look under the "services" tab for information on how to collect and send your specimen.

Dr. John Toth, DO
Cystitis Research Center
Advanced Integrative Medicine
2270 Bacon St., Concord CA 94520
(925) 687-9447

Pelvic Pain and Pelvic Floor Dysfunction

Books

Davies, C., and A. Davies. *The Trigger Point Therapy Workbook: Your Self-Treatment Guide for Pain Relief.* 2nd ed. Oakland, CA: New Harbinger Press, 2004.

Howard, F., C. Perry, J. Carter, et al. *Pelvic Pain Diagnosis and Management.* Philadelphia, PA: Lippincott Williams & Wilkins, 2000.

Stein, A. *Heal Pelvic Pain: A Proven Stretching, Strengthening, and Nutrition Program for Relieving Pain, Incontinence, IBS, and Other Symptoms Without Surgery.* New York: McGraw Hill, 2009.

Travell, J., and D. Simons. *The Trigger Point Manual*, Vol 2. Baltimore, MD: Williams and Wilkins, 1992.

Wise, D., and R. Anderson. *A Headache in the Pelvis: A New Understand-*

ing and Treatment for Prostatitis and Chronic Pelvic Pain Syndromes. Occidental, CA: National Center for Pelvic Pain, 2003.

Articles
Weiss, J. "Chronic Pelvic Pain and Myofascial Trigger Points." *The Pain Clinic* 2, no. 6 (December 2000):13–18.

Organizations, Support Groups, and Websites
American Urogynecology Society Foundation (AUGS)
www.mypelvichealth.org
Information about pelvic floor disorders (PFD), a treatable medical condition affecting millions of women. An excellent medical resource for a variety of pelvic health disorders.

Beyond Basics Physical Therapy
www.beyondbasicsphysicaltherapy.com
This is the website of Amy Stein, MPT, the author of Heal Pelvic Pain: A Proven Stretching, Strengthening, and Nutrition Program for Relieving Pain, Incontinence, IBS, and Other Symptoms Without Surgery *(cited above under book resources for Pelvic Pain). She practices in New York, NY.*

George Washington University Pelvic Floor Center
Washington DC
www.gwhospital.com/Hospital-Services-O-Z/Pelvic-Floor-Center /Pelvic-Floor-Doctors

Pelvic Health and Rehabilitation Center
San Francisco CA
www.pelvicpainrehab.com/about_us

The Wise-Anderson Protocol (formerly called The Stanford Protocol)
www.pelvicpainhelp.com
Learn all about this approach at this website.

Prostatitis and Chronic Prostatitis/Chronic Pelvic Pain Syndrome (CPPS)

Books
Davies, C., and A. Davies. *The Trigger Point Therapy Workbook: Your Self-Treatment Guide for Pain Relief.* 2nd ed. Oakland, CA: New Harbinger Press, 2004.

Murray, M., and J. Pizzorno. *Encyclopedia of Natural Medicine.* Rev. 2nd ed. New York: Three Rivers Press, 1998. *Good general information source on natural healing, herbs, and naturopathic medicine. I am in-cluding it here particularly for a good description of the use of herbs to treat benign enlargement of the prostate (BPH). See pages 753–62.*

Stein, A. *Heal Pelvic Pain: A Proven Stretching, Strengthening, and Nutrition Program for Relieving Pain, Incontinence, IBS, and Other Symptoms Without Surgery.* New York: McGraw Hill, 2009. *A good general reference, albeit covering a large territory. The author does include a short chapter "For Men Only" that discusses chronic prostatitis (see pages 153–56).*

Wise, D., and R. Anderson. *A Headache in the Pelvis: A New Understanding and Treatment for Prostatitis and Chronic Pelvic Pain Syndromes.* Occidental, CA: National Center for Pelvic Pain, 2003. *A good general discussion of men's chronic pelvic pain disorders. For prostatitis, see pages 31–40.*

Articles

Anderson, R., et al. "Sexual Dysfunction in Men with Chronic Prostatitis/Chronic Pelvic Pain Syndrome: Improvement after Trigger Point Release and Paradoxical Relaxation Training." *Journal of Urology* 176 (October 2005): 1534–38.

Anderson, W. "A Headache in the Pelvis: An Introduction to a New Pelvic Pain Therapy Program for IC, Prostatitis, Vulvodynia, and Other Related Conditions." *ICN Guest Lecture Series*, Stanford, CA, 8 July 2003. *For full text of discussion, see http://www.ic-network.com /guestlectures/anderson.html.*

Nickel, J., et al. "Prevalence of Prostatitis-Like Symptoms in a Population-Based Study Using the National Institutes of Health Chronic Prostatitis Symptom Index." *Journal of Urology* 165 (suppl) (2001): 23.

Organizations, Support Groups, and Websites

Harvard Medical College — Prostate Disease
www.harvardprostateknowledge.org/prostate-health-resources

International Pelvic Pain Society
www.pelvicpain.org

The National Center for Pelvic Pain Research (NCPPR)
www.pelvicpainhelp.com
The NCPPR is a center devoted to research and the treatment of pelvic pain syndromes in men and women using the Wise-Anderson (Stanford) Protocol.

The Prostatitis Foundation
www.prostatitis.org
Offers comprehensive information on prostate disorders.

The Urology Channel
www.urologychannel.com/prostate/prostatitis/index.shtml
Good explanation of prostatitis.

Vulvodynia

Books

Goldstein, A., C. Pukall, and I. Goldstein. *Female Sexual Pain Disorders: Evaluation and Management.* Hoboken, NJ: Wiley-Blackwell, 2009. *Apparently this is one of the few really good books on vulvodynia. It appears to be a comprehensive, scientific approach to intimate pain.*

Vliet, E. L. *Screaming to Be Heard: The Hormonal Connections Women Suspect and Doctors Still Ignore.* Rev. and exp. ed. New York: M. Evans and Company, 2001.

Articles

Boardman, L. A., A. S. Cooper, L. R. Blais, and C. A. Raker. "Topical Gabapentin in the Treatment of Localized and Generalized Vulvodynia." *Obstetrics and Gynecology* 112, no. 3 (September 2008): 579–85.

Reed, B. "Vulvodynia: Diagnosis and Management." *American Family Physician* 73 (2006): 1231–39. *This is a very comprehensive discussion of vulvodynia.*

Saldinger, A. G. "*Vulvar Pain Syndrome: You Are Not Alone.*" 1998, revised 23 January 2009, by Marlene M. Maheu. http://www.selfhelp magazine.com/article/node/1070. *Very informative and compassionate look at vulvodynia.*

Sutton, J. T., G. A. Bachmann, L. D. Arnold, G. G. Rhoads, and R. C. Rosen. "Assessment of Vulvodynia Symptoms in a Sample of U.S. Women: A Follow-up National Incidence Survey." *Journal of Women's Health* 17, no. 8 (1 October 2008): 1285–92.

Organizations, Support Groups, and Websites

American College of Obstetricians and Gynecologists (ACOG)
www.acog.org/publications/patient_education/bp127.cfm

The International Pelvic Pain Society (IPPS)
www.pelvicpain.org

National Vulvodynia Association (NVA)
(301) 299-0775   www.nva.org

Society for Women's Health
(202) 223-8224   info@womenshealthresearch.org

Vulvar Pain Foundation (VPF)
(910) 226-0704   www.vulvarpainfoundation.org

Vulval Pain Society (UK)
www.vulvalpainsociety.org

Overactive Bladder (OAB) and Incontinence

Books

Newman, D., and A. Wein. *Overcoming Overactive Bladder: Your Complete Self-Care Guide.* Oakland, CA: New Harbinger Publications, 2004. *One of the most readable books for the seventeen million people in the United States suffering from OAB, offering medical treatments and behavioral coping techniques.*

Rogers, R., and J. Shagam. *Regaining Bladder Control: What Every Woman Needs to Know.* Amherst, NY: Prometheus Books, 2006. *One of the more recent books on incontinence and OAB, for both professionals and patients.*

Articles

Mayo Clinic. "Urinary Incontinence." http://www.mayoclinic.com /health/urinary-incontinence/DS00404; "Overactive Bladder." http://www.mayoclinic.com/health/overactive-bladder/DS00827.

The Urology Channel. "Overview of Urinary Incontinence." http://www.urologychannel.com/incontinence/index.shtml; "Overactive Bladder Overview." http://www.urologychannel.com/bladdercontrol/index.shtml.

Web MD. "Treatment Options for Overactive Bladder." (reviewed by Marcel Horowitz, 21 September 2009). http://www.webmd.com /urinary-incontinence-oab/oab-8/oab-treatment.

Organizations, Support Groups, and Websites

Cystitis and Overactive Bladder Foundation (OAB online support group)
http://cobf.websitetoolbox.com

Daily Strength: Urinary Incontinence Online Support Group
www.dailystrength.org

National Association for Continence (NAFC)
www.nafc.org/bladder-bowel-health

The Simon Foundation for Continence
(800) 23-SIMON   www.simonfoundation.org

The Urology Channel — Bladder Control
www.urologychannel.com/bladdercontrol/index.shtml
Informative site for those with bladder control issues.

The Urology Channel — Incontinence
www.urologychannel.com/incontinence/index.shtml
Information on incontinence by The Urology Channel staff.

UrologyHealth.org
www.urologyhealth.org/adult/index.cfm?cat=03&topic=450&x=16&y=15
Good informational site on OAB and other urinary problems.

Web MD
www.webmd.com/urinary-incontinence-oab/oab-8/oab-treatment
Information and resource referral for OAB and incontinence.

General Urological Information

Organizations, Support Groups, and Websites

American Urological Association (AUA)
(410) 727-1100   www.auanet.org   aua@auanet.org

American Urological Association Foundation (AUAF)
www.urologyhealth.org

American Urogynecologic Society (AUGS)
www.augs.org

National Kidney and Urologic Diseases Information Clearinghouse
3 Information Way, Bethesda MD 20892-3580
(800) 891-5390   nkudic@info.niddk.nih.gov
www.kidney.niddk.nih.gov

WellBladder.com
www.wellbladder.com
The author's website.

Gluten Intolerance and Celiac Disease

Books

Braly, J., and R. Hoggan. *Dangerous Grains: Why Gluten Cereal Grains May Be Hazardous to Your Health.* New York: Avery/Penguin, 2002.

Cohan, W. *Gluten-Free Portland: A Resource Guide.* Self-published bian-nually. *Comprehensive guide to the gluten-free diet, written by the author of this book.* Books can be ordered through the author's website: www.glutenfreechoice.com.

Green, P. H. R., and R. Jones. *Celiac Disease: A Hidden Epidemic.* New York: William Morrow, 2006. *Written by the director of the Celiac Disease Center at Columbia University. This book was recently updated and rereleased (2010).*

Libonati, C. J. *Recognizing Celiac Disease: Signs, Symptoms, Associated Disorders, and Complications.* Fort Washington, PA: Gluten Free Works Publishing, 2007. *A comprehensive clinical guide to celiac and non-celiac gluten intolerance symptoms and pathology.*

Lieberman, S., with L. Segall. *The Gluten Connection: How Gluten Sensitivity May Be Sabotaging Your Health — And What You Can Do to Take Control NOW.* New York: Rodale Press, 2007.

Wangen, S. *Healthier Without Wheat: A New Understanding of Wheat Allergies, Celiac Disease, and Non-Celiac Gluten Intolerance.* Seattle, WA: Innate Health Publishing, 2009.

Articles

Fasano, A. "Medicine Man: Alessio Fasano, MD, Is Making Big Strides for Celiac Disease." *Living Without* (June/July 2008).

Fasano, A. "Celiac Disease: How to Handle a Clinical Chameleon." *New England Journal of Medicine* 348 (19 June 2003): 2568–79.

Helms, S. "Celiac Disease and Gluten-Associated Diseases." *Alternative Medicine Review* 10, no. 3 (2005): 172–92.

Nelsen, D. "Gluten-Sensitive Enteropathy (Celiac Disease): More Common Than You Think." *American Family Physician* 66, no. 12 (15 December 2002): 2259–66.

Organizations, Support Groups, and Websites

Canadian Celiac Association (CCA)

(800) 363-7296   celiac@look.ca   www.celiac.ca

Celiac Disease Foundation (CDF)

(818) 990-2354   cdf@celiac.org   www.celiac.org
Provides education and outreach.

Celiac Information and Support

www.celiac.com
Scott Adams has a very helpful and comprehensive website on gluten intol-

erance—great recipes, monthly newsletter, blog, articles, and a large database of previously published articles.

Celiac Sprue Association

(402) 558-0600   celiacs@csaceliacs.org   www.csaceliacs.org

Enterolab

10875 Plano Rd., Ste. 123, Dallas TX 75238

(972) 686-6869   www.enterolab.com

Provides stool testing for antibodies indicating presence of celiac disease or gluten intolerance.

Gluten Free Choice

www.glutenfreechoice.com

The author's website on gluten intolerance, including informative articles discussing the link between celiac disease, gluten intolerance, and bladder symptoms, including IC.

Gluten Intolerance Group (GIG)

(206) 246-6652   info@gluten.net   www.gluten.net

Has local branches in communities nationwide, and sponsors a national education conference annually.

National Digestive Diseases Information Clearinghouse (NDDIC)

http://digestive.niddk.nih.gov

Prometheus Laboratories Inc.

9410 Carroll Park Dr., San Diego CA 92121

(888) 423-5227, opt. #3   www.prometheuslabs.com

Provides testing for celiac disease and gluten intolerance.

Gluten-Free Diet

Books

Case, S. *Gluten-Free Diet: A Comprehensive Resource Guide.* Rev. and exp. ed. Regina, Saskatchewan: Case Nutritional Consulting, 2008.

O'Brien, S. *Gluten-free, Sugar-free Cooking: Over 200 Delicious Recipes to Help You Live a Healthier, Allergy-Free Life.* Portland, OR: Marlowe & Company, 2006.

Robertson, K. *Cooking Gluten-Free! A Food Lover's Collection of Chef and Family Recipes Without Gluten or Wheat.* Seattle, WA: Celiac Publishing, 2002.

Shepherd, J. *The First Year: Celiac Disease and Living Gluten-Free: An Essential Guide for the Newly Diagnosed.* New York: DaCapo Press, 2008.

Healthy Diet Resources

Books

Black, J. *The Anti-Inflammation Diet and Recipe Book: Protect Yourself and Your Family from Heart Disease, Arthritis, Diabetes, Allergies—and More*. Alameda, CA: Hunter House Publishers, 2006.

Bundy, A. *Sweet Alternatives: More than 100 Recipes Without Gluten, Dairy, and Soy*. Vancouver, BC: Whitecap, 2005.

Campbell, T. C., and T. M. Campbell II. *The China Study: Startling Implications for Diet, Weight Loss and Long-term Health*. Dallas, TX: Benbella Books, 2006.

Catalano, A. *Baking with Agave Nectar: Over 100 Recipes Using Nature's Ultimate Sweetener*. Berkeley, CA: Celestial Arts, 2008.

Cordain, L. *The Paleo Diet: Lose Weight and Get Healthy by Eating the Food You Were Designed to Eat*. Hoboken, NJ: John Wiley & Sons, 2002.

Crook, W. G. *The Yeast Connection Handbook: How Yeasts Can Make You Feel "Sick All Over" and the Steps You Need to Take to Regain Your Health*. Garden City Park, NY: Square One Publishers, 1999.

Freed, D. L. "Dietary Lectins and Disease." In *Food Allergy and Intolerance*, ed. by J. Brostoff and S. J. Challacombe. London: Bailliere Tindall, 1987.

Marti, J. M., and Z. P. Rona. *Complete Candida Yeast Guidebook: Everything You Need to Know About Prevention, Treatment and Diet*. Rev. 2nd ed. New York: Three Rivers Press, 2000.

Vasey, C. *The Acid-Alkaline Diet for Optimum Health: Restore Your Health by Creating pH Balance in Your Diet*. Rev. 2nd ed. Rochester, VT: Healing Arts Press, 2006.

Winderlin, C., with K. Sennert. *Candida-Related Complex: What Your Doctor Might Be Missing*. Boulder, CO: Taylor Trade Publishing, 1996.

Organizations, Support Groups, and Websites

International Chronic Urticaria Society
www.urticaria.thunderworksinc.com/pages/lowhistamine.htm
Provides comprehensive food lists for low-histamine diet.

Rowan's Resources
www.branwen.com/rowan/oxalate.htm
Information provided by a patient on following a low histamine diet.

University of Pittsburg Medical Center (UPMC)
www.upmc.com/HealthAtoZ/Pages/HealthLibrary.aspx?chunkiid=196214
Provides information for consumers on how to follow a low-histamine diet.

Articles (and Newsletters)
Nutrition Action Newsletter — The Center for Science in the Public Interest
www.cspinet.org/nah
Practical nutritional advice for consumers.

The Harvard Women's Health Watch Newsletter
www.health.harvard.edu
Sign up for this free newsletter.

Sullivan, K. "The Lectin Report."
http://www.krispin.com/lectin.html
Good introductory article on lectins.

Menopause and Hormonal Imbalances

Books
Martin, M., and J. Gerstung. *The Estrogen Alternative: A Guide to Natural Hormonal Balance.* 4th ed. Rochester, VT: Healing Arts Press, 2005. *Although this book may now be somewhat outdated with regard to hormone replacement therapy, it is a very comprehensive guide to natural hormone balance and includes important discussions on hormones and osteoporosis and cancer. The authors favor natural progesterone supplementation.*

Northrup, C. *The Wisdom of Menopause: Creating Physical and Emotional Health During the Change.* Rev. ed. New York: Bantam Books, 2006.

Northrup, C. *Women's Bodies, Women's Wisdom: Creating Physical and Emotional Health and Healing.* New York: Bantam Books, 2006.

Vliet, E. L. *Screaming to Be Heard: The Hormonal Connections Women Suspect and Doctors Still Ignore.* Rev. and exp. ed. New York: M. Evans and Company, 2001.

Author's Note: I particularly recommend Dr. Northrup's and Dr. Vliet's books. These are traditional allopathic physicians with open minds and a deep understanding of holistic medicine. In addition, I respect the way they keep up on the latest science and apply it to their treatment approaches, even when this requires a significant change of paradigm.

Organizations, Support Groups, and Websites
Christiane Northrup, MD
www.drnorthrup.com
Interactive website on women's health.

Natural Woman Institute (NWI)
www.naturalwoman.org
National database of medical practitioners specializing in natural, bioidentical hormone treatment.

For Children

Books
Author's Note: *The Better Bladder Book* deals primarily with adult health problems, so information provided for children here is limited. I do highly recommend reading the article on food sensitivities in children, cited here and also accessible via the link on my website, www.wellbladder.com. For more assistance, contact the pediatric-specialty resources below.

Articles
Alpha Online. http://www.nutramed.com/children/children_bladder_kidneys.htm. *Excellent article on food sensitivities and bladder problems in children.*

Organizations, Support Groups, and Websites
Division of Pediatric Urology
The Brady Urological Institute
Johns Hopkins Hospital
Baltimore, MD
http://urology.jhu.edu/pediatric

Pediatric Urology Clinic at Lucile Packard Children's Hospital
Stanford University, CA
www.lpch.org/clinicalSpecialtiesServices/ClinicalSpecialties/Urology/urologyClinic.html

The Society for Pediatric Urology
www.spuonline.org

Complementary/Integrative Therapies

Books
Dossey, L. *Healing Words: The Power of Prayer and the Practice of Medicine.* New York: HarperCollins, 1993.

Jahnke, R. *The Healer Within: Using Traditional Chinese Techniques to Release Your Body's Own Medicine.* San Francisco, CA: HarperCollins, 1999.

Weiselfish-Giammatteo, S. *Body Wisdom: Light Touch for Optimal Health*. Berkeley, CA: North Atlantic Books, 2002. *Best source for more information on the techniques of Integrative Manual Therapy (IMT) and Neurofascial Processing (NFP).*

Organizations, Support Groups, and Websites

American Association of Oriental Medicine (AAOM)
(866) 455-7999   www.aaom.org
Offers referrals for acupuncturists in your community.

American Holistic Medical Association (AHMA)
www.holisticmedicine.org
National database listing physicians from a variety of specialties. An online referral service and a guide to finding a holistic practitioner in your community.

CenterIMT [Integrative Medicine]
www.centerimt.com/home.asp

Healthandgoodness.com
www.healthandgoodness.com/Therapies/IMT-session.html

Integrative Manual Therapy Association
www.imtassociation.org

National Center for Complementary and Alternative Medicine
http://nccam.nih.gov/nccam

Centers for IC Research

The Interstitial Cystitis Clinical Research Network (ICCRN) is made up of ten clinical centers and a central data-coordinating center. This network was set up to conduct clinical trials to evaluate various therapies for IC. Because there are many similarities with research design and clinical treatment of chronic prostatitis, the former Chronic Prostatitis Collaborative Research Network (CPCRN) also participates in common research under the umbrella of the Urological Pelvic Pain Collaborative Research Network (UPPCRN). If you are near one of the centers listed below, it may be possible for you to participate in a clinical trial. These centers are also likely to be a good source for referrals to specialists treating IC in your area.

California
Stanford University Medical Center, Palo Alto CA
(650) 724-1753

Canada
Queen's University, Kingston, Ontario
(613) 533-2894

Illinois
Loyola University Medical Center, Maywood IL
(708) 216-8495

Iowa
University of Iowa, Iowa City IA
(319) 384-9265

Maryland
University of Maryland, Baltimore MD
(410) 328-5108

Massachusetts
Tufts University School of Medicine, New England Medical Center, Boston
(617) 636-6317

Michigan
Henry Ford Hospital, Detroit MI
(313) 916-8972

William Beaumont Hospital, Royal Oak MI
(248) 551-0885

New York
University of Rochester, Rochester NY
(585) 275-0133

Pennsylvania
University of Pennsylvania, Philadelphia PA
(215) 615-3780

Washington
University of Washington, Seattle WA
(206) 598-6357

Index